Joint U.S.-Mexico Workshop on Preventing Obesity in Children and Youth of Mexican Origin

SUMMARY

Maria Oria and Kristin Sawyer, *Rapporteurs*

Food and Nutrition Board

INSTITUTE OF MEDICINE
OF THE NATIONAL ACADEMIES

THE NATIONAL ACADEMIES PRESS
Washington, D.C.
www.nap.edu

THE NATIONAL ACADEMIES PRESS 500 Fifth STREET, N.W. Washington, DC 20001

NOTICE: The project that is the subject of this report was approved by the Governing Board of the National Research Council, whose members are drawn from the councils of the National Academy of Sciences, the National Academy of Engineering, and the Institute of Medicine. The members of the committee responsible for the report were chosen for their special competences and with regard for appropriate balance.

The activity was supported by a grant between the National Academy of Sciences and Kaiser Permanente. Any opinions, findings, conclusions, or recommendations expressed in this publication are those of the authors and do not necessarily reflect the views of the organizations or agencies that provided support for the project.

International Standard Book Number-13: 978-0-309-10325-1
International Standard Book Number-10: 0-309-10325-8

Additional copies of this report are available from the National Academies Press, 500 Fifth Street, N.W., Lockbox 285, Washington, DC 20055; (800) 624-6242 or (202) 334-3313 (in the Washington metropolitan area); Internet, http://www.nap.edu.

For more information about the Institute of Medicine, visit the IOM home page at: **www.iom.edu.**

Printed in the United States of America.

The serpent has been a symbol of long life, healing, and knowledge among almost all cultures and religions since the beginning of recorded history. The serpent adopted as a logotype by the Institute of Medicine is a relief carving from ancient Greece, now held by the Staatliche Museen in Berlin.

"Knowing is not enough; we must apply.
Willing is not enough; we must do."
—Goethe

INSTITUTE OF MEDICINE
OF THE NATIONAL ACADEMIES

Advising the Nation. Improving Health.

THE NATIONAL ACADEMIES

Advisers to the Nation on Science, Engineering, and Medicine

The **National Academy of Sciences** is a private, nonprofit, self-perpetuating society of distinguished scholars engaged in scientific and engineering research, dedicated to the furtherance of science and technology and to their use for the general welfare. Upon the authority of the charter granted to it by the Congress in 1863, the Academy has a mandate that requires it to advise the federal government on scientific and technical matters. Dr. Ralph J. Cicerone is president of the National Academy of Sciences.

The **National Academy of Engineering** was established in 1964, under the charter of the National Academy of Sciences, as a parallel organization of outstanding engineers. It is autonomous in its administration and in the selection of its members, sharing with the National Academy of Sciences the responsibility for advising the federal government. The National Academy of Engineering also sponsors engineering programs aimed at meeting national needs, encourages education and research, and recognizes the superior achievements of engineers. Dr. Wm. A. Wulf is president of the National Academy of Engineering.

The **Institute of Medicine** was established in 1970 by the National Academy of Sciences to secure the services of eminent members of appropriate professions in the examination of policy matters pertaining to the health of the public. The Institute acts under the responsibility given to the National Academy of Sciences by its congressional charter to be an adviser to the federal government and, upon its own initiative, to identify issues of medical care, research, and education. Dr. Harvey V. Fineberg is president of the Institute of Medicine.

The **National Research Council** was organized by the National Academy of Sciences in 1916 to associate the broad community of science and technology with the Academy's purposes of furthering knowledge and advising the federal government. Functioning in accordance with general policies determined by the Academy, the Council has become the principal operating agency of both the National Academy of Sciences and the National Academy of Engineering in providing services to the government, the public, and the scientific and engineering communities. The Council is administered jointly by both Academies and the Institute of Medicine. Dr. Ralph J. Cicerone and Dr. Wm. A. Wulf are chair and vice chair, respectively, of the National Research Council.

www.national-academies.org

PLANNING COMMITTEE ON JOINT U.S.–MEXICO WORKSHOP ON PREVENTING OBESITY OF CHILDREN AND YOUTH OF MEXICAN ORIGIN

REYNALDO MARTORELL (*Chair*), Hubert Department of Global Health, Rollins School of Public Health, Emory University, Atlanta, GA
JEFFREY KOPLAN, Woodruff Health Sciences Center, Emory University, Atlanta, GA
JUAN RIVERA, National Institutes of Public Health, Morelos, México

Consultant Writers

SIMÓN BARQUERA, Research Center for Nutrition and Health, Morelos, México
BERNARDO HERNÁNDEZ, Research Center for Population Health: Reproductive Health Division, Morelos, México
RUY LÓPEZ, Research Center for Population Health: Chronic Disease Division, Morelos, México
FERNANDO MENDOZA, Stanford University School of Medicine, Palo Alto, CA
JUAN RIVERA, Research Center for Nutrition and Health, Morelos, México
FREDERICK TROWBRIDGE, Trowbridge & Associates, Inc., Atlanta, GA

Staff

MARIA ORIA, Study Director
VIVICA KRAAK, Study Director (until February 2006)
LINDA D. MEYERS, Director, Food and Nutrition Board
SANDRA AMAMOO-KAKRA, Senior Program Assistant
JON SANDERS, Senior Program Assistant (until June 2006)

FOOD AND NUTRITION BOARD*

*IOM Boards do not review or approve individual reports and are not asked to endorse conclusions and recommendations. The responsibility for the content of the report rests with the authoring committee and the institution.

Reviewers

This report has been reviewed in draft form by individuals chosen for their diverse perspectives and technical expertise, in accordance with procedures approved by the NRC's Report Review Committee. The purpose of this independent review is to provide candid and critical comments that will assist the institution in making its published report as sound as possible and to ensure that the report meets institutional standards for objectivity, evidence, and responsiveness to the study charge. The review comments and draft manuscript remain confidential to protect the integrity of the deliberative process. We wish to thank the following individuals for their review of this report:

George R. Flores, The California Endowment, San Francisco, CA
Amy Luke, Loyola University School of Medicine, Chicago, IL
Roberto Medina-Santillán, Mexican Academy of Medicine, México D.F.
Roberto Otto Valdez, Valdez and Associates, Vienna, VA

Although the reviewers listed above have provided many constructive comments and suggestions, they were not asked to endorse the final draft of the summary before its release. The review of this report was overseen by **Eileen Kennedy** of Tufts University. Appointed by the National Research Council and Institute of Medicine, she was responsible for making certain that an independent examination of this report was carried out in accordance with institutional procedures and that all review comments were carefully considered. Responsibility for the final content of this report rests entirely with the authoring committee and the institution.

Preface

Moved by the alarming findings in the Institute of Medicine (IOM) report *Preventing Childhood Obesity: Health in the Balance* (2005), which addresses the high prevalence in obesity among the Hispanic population, and motivated by follow-up discussions among members of the IOM's Food and Nutrition Board (FNB) and the Committee on Prevention of Obesity in Children and Youth, IOM formed a planning committee to plan a workshop that would increase understanding of the obesity epidemic among Mexican and Mexican–American children and youth in the United States and Mexico. Three reasons for focusing on Mexicans on both sides of the border were the gravity of the obesity problem among Mexicans in both countries; the large population sizes involved (e.g., Mexicans are the majority of the Hispanic population in the United States); and finally, the fact that the two countries share common cultural, dietary, environmental, and economic characteristics. An early assumption was that it makes sense for the United States and Mexico to share lessons and experiences related to the obesity problem.

The Instituto Nacional de la Salud Pública (INSP) in Mexico—a public health institution that seeks to redress social and health inequity through research and educational programs—was instrumental in identifying the nature of this cooperative effort and its objectives. Initial discussion on the appropriate structure for a possible meeting led to the development of a two-day workshop in which selected Mexican and U.S. leaders from government, foundations, nongovernmental organizations, academia, the food industry, and media would participate. The format of the workshop was planned to stimulate dialogue and discussion through small group and plenary discussions.

As chair of the planning committee, I would like to extend a special thanks to Mauricio Hernández, Director General of INSP, for his continued support and willingness to host the workshop at INSP headquarters. My sincere thanks also go to the other two members of the planning committee: Juan Rivera, Director of the Centro de Investigación en Nutrición y Salud, INSP, and Jeffrey Koplan, Vice President for Academic Health Affairs, the Woodruff Health Sciences Center of Emory University. Their leadership and contributions throughout the planning period and during the workshop were invaluable. INSP's Ruy Lopez, Simon Barquera, and Bernardo Hernández were helpful in identifying key topics and issues relevant to the Mexican context—a difficult task when there are many unknowns and a general lack of awareness regarding Mexico's obesity epidemic. In addition, they played a central role in identifying and inviting workshop participants who brought important insights into the prevalence of obesity, on developing interventions, and future opportunities in Mexico.

Many thanks to the authors of the two thorough reviews that were commissioned to provide a background about the childhood obesity problem in Mexico (Juan Rivera, Ruy Lopez, Simon Barquera, and Bernardo Hernández) and in the United States (Frederick Trowbridge, from Trowbridge and Associates, Inc., and Fernando Mendoza from Stanford University's School of Medicine). The authors not only offered a comprehensive picture of the epidemic but also provided insightful presentations. The presentations and group and panel discussions generated stimulating perspectives among participants. More importantly, they served as a platform for discussion focused on the ultimate goal—the feasibility of a binational program to prevent obesity in children of Mexican origin. Sincere thanks go to all the presenters, rapporteurs, and panel presenters. It was an honor to have in the audience such distinguished speakers as Jaime Sepúlveda, Coordinator of the Institutos Nacionales de Salud at the Mexican Ministry of Health, and Julio Frenk, Mexican Minister of Health. I also would like to extend my gratitude to all workshop participants, whose contributions made this event such a rich experience.

I would like to thank Kaiser Permanente, financial supporter of the project, and its representatives at the meeting: Diana Bonta and Esteban Cruz. Finally, thanks to Linda Meyers, Maria Oria, Vivica Kraak, Jon Sanders, and Sandra Amamoo-Kakra from IOM/FNB and Juan Manuel Irizas from INSP for their dedication and their efforts in making this workshop a successful one.

It is my hope that this workshop is only a first step toward the common goal of reversing the increasing prevalence of childhood obesity and preventing the onset of associated chronic diseases. Future collaborative activities (with Mexico or other countries) certainly will follow.

Reynaldo Martorell, *Chair*
Chair, Planning Committee

Contents

Summary

Over the past two decades, there has been an alarming, unprecedented increase in childhood and adolescent obesity and at-risk-of obesity[1] that has reached epidemic proportions. This increase has raised worldwide awareness and concern, particularly regarding the link between obesity and serious, chronic health conditions like diabetes, cardiovascular disease, hyperlipidemia, and others. The ultimate solution for reversing obesity requires maintaining energy balance and a healthy lifestyle; such a solution implies the development and implementation of specific, feasible, and efficient strategies and interventions defined through political, social, and cultural contexts specific for each country.

The Institute of Medicine (IOM) report *Preventing Childhood Obesity: Health in the Balance* (2005) found that among U.S. children, those of Hispanic origin, especially Mexican–American children, have the highest rates of obesity. Moreover, the obesity epidemic has been recognized in Mexico as well, where the public health community is paying increased attention to survey data indicating the growing obesity rates among children, youth, and adults. These findings, as well as the recognition of the unique context of the Mexican–American population in the United States

[1]Obese children or youth refers to those with age- and gender-specific body mass index (BMI) that is equal to or greater than the 95th percentile of the Centers for Disease Control and Prevention (CDC) BMI charts. Children and youth at-risk for obesity are those with BMI-for-age 85th percentile to less than 95th percentile.

and the many similarities shared between the United States and Mexico, served as the basis for the initial discussions that resulted in this workshop.

Since the 1500s Mexican Americans have lived in what is now the southwestern United States and have maintained a continuing cultural and commercial exchange with Mexico. In fact, Mexicans continue to immigrate to the United States in unprecedented numbers. As they integrate in American society, they maintain their culture but also begin a process of acculturation, that is, they adopt many social norms and habits of the United States, including those related to diet and exercise; the consequences of acculturation in obesity prevalence are intriguing and still unclear.

Although, as already mentioned, solutions to prevent obesity should be feasible within the specific context of each country, the substantial and ongoing interchange of people and culture between the United States and Mexico necessitates an obesity prevention approach that recognizes the common social, cultural, and economic factors that contribute to childhood obesity in both countries. With this in mind, the IOM, with the Instituto Nacional de la Salud Pública (INSP) and supported by Kaiser Permanente, sponsored a joint U.S.–Mexico workshop that involved researchers, public health officials, industry leaders, and policy makers from both sides of the border. The primary objective of the workshop was to explore the potential for a U.S.–Mexico binational obesity prevention strategy by considering the perspectives and experiences of various stakeholders—governments, research institutions, industry, non-governmental organizations, and communities. Other objectives included assessing similarities and differences in the prevention of obesity in Mexican and Mexican–American children, sharing policy and program experiences, and identifying data and information gaps. This workshop summary focuses on the nature of childhood obesity, its magnitude and distribution, current and future policies and programs, and data needs. This summary should not be perceived as a series of recommendations reached by consensus but rather as a recapitulation of the discussions of speakers, working groups, and individual participants.

As background for the workshop, two papers were commissioned. The first paper, "Preventing Obesity in Mexican Children and Adolescents," reviews the factors that contribute to the high obesity prevalence in Mexican children and adolescents, provides an overview of current obesity intervention programs, and proposes actions to prevent the epidemic. A second paper, "Preventing Obesity in Mexican–American Children and Adolescents," addresses similar topics from a U.S. perspective.

OBESITY PREVALENCE AND ASSOCIATED FACTORS IN PEOPLE OF MEXICAN ORIGIN

Preventing Childhood Obesity: Health in the Balance (IOM, 2005) included an ecological model of the obesity problem and recommendations for action to all stakeholders. In the United States, CDC data demonstrated an alarming growth in obesity prevalence—among U.S. children and adolescents the rate tripled from approximately 5 percent to about 16 percent within the last 40 years. In Mexico, the data available from the National Nutrition Surveys show an increase of more than 30 percent from the 1988 to the 1999 survey in at-risk for obesity and obese Mexican children 2–4 years old. The 1999 survey indicates a high prevalence (16 percent) of obesity and at-risk of obesity among Mexican children, occurring in all regions, rural and urban areas, and in both girls and boys ages 2–17 years. At substantially higher levels, the obesity and at-risk for obesity prevalence among Mexican–American boys 2–11 years of age is about 38 percent. The epidemiological data presented show the existence of an obesity epidemic in Mexico with similar characteristics to the one in the United States.

This continued increase in prevalence makes obesity a problem of epidemic proportions, with a behavior that is comparable to the characteristics of infectious diseases. The negative implications of this rising trend in obesity for the economy and health on both sides of the border call for an urgent prevention strategy on all fronts.

Many factors associated with the risk of obesity are complex, including psychosocial, dietary, and physical activity factors, which ultimately are related to energy balance—the fundamental issue underlying the epidemic. As an example, changes in the diets are occurring in people on both sides of the border. Data presented show that instead of selecting fruits and vegetables in their diets, Mexicans as well as Mexican Americans are choosing more high-energy, less-nutritious foods. In Mexico, this might be related to cost, urbanization, changes in family structures, or other social factors. In the United States, on the other hand, the process of acculturation to the U.S. social rules and habits might be a contributor to the increasing obesity prevalence. Differences in the nature and occurrence of these nutritional transitions may explain one notable difference between the United States and Mexico—the relationship between socioeconomic status (SES) and the prevalence of obesity. In Mexico, a higher SES is associated with a higher prevalence of obesity, whereas the opposite relationship prevails in the United States. The relationships between obesity and SES in both countries might be simply explained by a difference in the progression of the epidemic in both countries that is, dietary changes experienced in both countries at different times, rather than a reflection of differences in dietary risk factors.

On the other side of the equation, data from physical activity tendencies call to the need for changes in this area. Data point to a low level of physical activity during and after school and a concurrent increasing trend in screen-viewing activities among children and youth in Mexico and the United States. This increase in sedentary activities might be spurred by a combination of factors related to safety concerns, lack of resources and time in schools, expense of activities, or other factors. In addition, having and enjoying appliances like televisions, computers, and cars provide a certain social status, therefore, supporting the hypothesis that a high SES might be causing a more obesigenic lifestyle.

Other cultural factors that are unique to the Hispanic population and define Mexicans on both sides of the border include the perception that being plump is equated with being at a healthy weight, and adherence to values that favor family needs over personal ones.

RESEARCH AND INFORMATION GAPS

Critical information gaps that thwart progress in obesity prevention among children and youth still remain and include the following two main themes: (1) risk factors leading to childhood obesity, particularly those related to behavioral patterns, along with strategies for interventions and implementations, and (2) design and implementation of studies to evaluate the efficacy of interventions and programs. Concerted efforts need to be directed towards solution-oriented research—research designs that lead directly to policy or practice changes that also include an evaluation component—in various areas; industry participation was seen as a necessity in translating research findings into effective interventions and programs.

Identifying Risk Factors and Developing Interventions and Implementation Strategies

What interventions and strategies will be effective in obesity prevention among Mexican–American and Mexican children? How should interventions be implemented? What specific intervention designs and testing are needed? Understanding behavioral factors through conducting experimental behavioral research on motivation and eating behaviors is critical to develop interventions that will result in long-term food and physical activity attitude changes. For example, searching for incentives to moderate the negative effects of acculturation and of adherence to certain values is an important focus of behavioral research. Another element of consumer behavior essential to designing effective interventions is that which derives from analysis of consumer responses to voluntary industry changes (e.g., new products and packaging). The industry could assist greatly in this endeavor by finding a mechanism for sharing marketing data; this is an area that was identified by individual participants as a current challenge.

To further assist in the design of randomized control trials on behavioral studies, researchers could conduct feasibility studies or pilot studies to test intervention strategies and identify potential barriers and facilitators of behavioral changes; this approach will help design and test appropriate intervention strategies before the more costly randomized control trials.

Information on other obesity-linked risk factors is scarce, so interventions are developed based on suggested associations. Therefore, there is a need to collect more data on obesity risk factors so that recommendations on interventions are based on sufficient evidence. For example, research on the effects of dietary content, eating patterns, physical activity and inactivity levels, and patterns leading to obesity prevention and weight control in already obese children could continue to be investigated so that a clearer picture of the factors and relationships among them can emerge. Once there is more evidence supporting the association between specific risk factors and obesity then a much broader testing of these interventions can be conducted in real-life scenarios.

Evaluating Interventions and Programs

An important aspect of reversing the obesity epidemic through interventions is evaluating programs that already have been implemented, internationally as well as locally. Researchers could gain important knowledge from those experiences and apply that knowledge to the development of new or improved strategies.

Much of the workshop participants' discussion focused on the importance of conducting studies for evaluating macro level interventions (e.g., evaluation of governmental policies and actions such as food and nutrition regulations, taxations, trade policies, urban planning policies, dietary and physical activity guidelines, or other current public health initiatives).

OBESITY PREVENTION SOLUTIONS

Participants conveyed the urgency of the situation and that, despite the dearth of data available to indisputably link risk factors to childhood obesity, key players have a responsibility to develop and implement strategies to prevent childhood obesity based on the best available evidence.

Role of Various Sectors

In general, the majority of participants found that the main premise for an obesity prevention strategy is that the causes of obesity follow an ecologic causal model, and therefore the strategy to mitigate the epidemic should be multilevel, multisectorial, and multidisciplinary. Some participants suggested that a cost-effectiveness analysis of the obesity epidemic is critical in helping decision makers prioritize resource allocation for health programs. As mentioned previously, interventions will need to be based on the best available evidence. If possible, using information from data on evaluation of the efficacy of interventions could be used as an important component of decision making.

Several workshop participants presented their perspectives and experiences on the role of the community, schools, industry, and government in implementing efficient prevention measures (see highlights in Box S-1). Discussions also highlighted differences in the countries' social and political systems and culture that could result in variations in implementation strategies.

Among the different perspectives presented, the issue of industry self-regulation versus government regulation to restrict food industry activities directed to children (e.g., marketing) was controversial. Ultimately, the group felt that industry self-regulation and government regulation both should be considered. The unifying theme in the group was that collaboration among sectors and disciplines is a crucial element of obesity prevention programs.

Next Steps Suggested by Working Groups and Individual Participants

Participants identified several barriers that are unique to the social and political context of each country. Ideas were discussed to overcome those barriers, and one major suggestion by Working Group III was the establishment of a government-led Mexican National Obesity Prevention Task Force paralleled to a joint U.S.–Mexico collaboration. Activities that could be the responsibility of this Mexican task force that were discussed by individual participants during the plenary are in Box S-2. Working Group III also proposed the creation of a U.S.–Mexico Obesity Prevention Task Force to initiate a collaboration to prevent obesity among children of Mexican heritage. Potential elements of such a collaboration are included in Box S-3 as summarized by Working Group III and discussed by individual participants in the plenary session. According to Working Group III, the responsibilities of the U.S.–Mexico Task Force would be the following:

- Develop a strategy to prevent obesity.
- Promote an obesity agenda with a specific timeline and responsibilities.
- Promote policies and norms that will allow environmental modifications in schools, worksites, cities, and other venues.
- Develop an educational strategy.

BOX S-1 The Role of Public and Private Sectors in Preventing Obesity

The following are perspectives on the role of various sectors in preventing obesity as viewed by panelists from Mexico and the United States.

Community (U.S. perspective)

- Many initiatives, including those to address health, originate from community-supported, social, nongovernmental, or consumer organizations.
- Changes in behavior will happen only when the community is involved in building healthier environments.
- Youth should contribute with their energy, ideas, and participation as an invaluable influence for community change and decision making.
- Resources to involve the community include
  - o Tools to educate the community on obesity as well as organizational and communication skills.
  - o Promotoras, as critical builders of trust between community members and authorities.
  - o Regular meetings with the city council or the local health department.

In Mexico, a sector that represents consumers' interests does not exist, and efforts in developing prevention strategies that involve community participation should be pursued by empowering the communities and encouraging advocacy activities.

Schools (Mexican perspective)

- Schools were seen as playing a pivotal role as an institution where interventions could have significant, long-term health benefits.
- The national physical education program should be viewed as an opportunity for implementing programs as advised by authoritative public health institutions.
- Some preventive actions are being implemented by improving nutrition and daily physical activity.
- Barriers to an obesity prevention strategy in schools are
  - o Lack of education programs on preventing obesity for children as well as for teachers and the general public.
  - o Insufficient nutrition information in school programs.
  - o Lack of resources (e.g., facilities) and time for physical activity programs.

continued

BOX S-1 Continued

Industry (U.S. and Mexican Perspective)

- The food industry has a definitive role in preventing obesity by
  - Providing a broader range of healthier products.
  - Informing the public on nutrition.
  - Forming alliances to support improvements in the quality and quantity of physical activities.
  - Collaborating on media educational campaigns, policy changes, and environmental changes.
- Self-regulating measures taken by industry might be effective but they include challenges, for instance the commitment of small companies.
- Other industries (e.g., electronics and communications) also need to be involved in obesity prevention programs and can contribute substantially to disseminating health messages.

Government (U.S. and Mexican Perspective)

- As a U.S. public health institution, the CDC has a role in research and disease surveillance, information dissemination, and public policy.
- Current approaches to obesity include prevention and control interventions.
- Collaboration with other institutions is critical in several areas, such as
  - Evaluating interventions that prevent and control obesity, and
  - Establishing indicators of obesity and implementing interventions.
- Mexican government programs for health promotion to prevent chronic diseases need improvement.
- Mexico needs a public health system that includes development, implementation, and enforcement of regulations as well as the power of litigation, especially for children.
- Such a regulatory process needs to be followed in a responsible manner, should be based on scientific findings and should consider the unique Mexican societal characteristics.

BOX S-2 Mexican National Obesity Prevention Task Force

Participants in Working Group III listed several elements for a Mexican National Obesity Prevention Task Force. These were further expanded by individual participants and include:

- **Increase the awareness.** By using survey data on prevalence of obesity, comorbidities, and cost estimates of the obesity epidemic, a coordinated effort from the medical and public health community, media, and government could raise awareness among the general public, medical community, government, and other decision makers.
- **Conduct assessment of human resources.** New public health challenges call for a careful assessment of human resources needs in areas such as research evaluation, intervention efficacy, and program management and implementation. The United States needs to continue developing those capabilities and can also play an important role in providing assistance.
- **Develop and implement a national policy for obesity prevention.** A national policy that ensures its continuation regardless of the changes in government is needed. This policy could draw from effective programs already implemented, with highest consideration given to the Mexican political, social, and cultural context.
- **Increase the participation of the community sector.** Educating and organizing the public is a critical effort that could provide the community with the important role they could play in advocacy and in imparting positive change by being active members of the community and participating in the decision-making process.
- **Build trust among various sectors.** Collaboration and trust among sectors is a very important step toward making progress to reverse the obesity epidemic. A model for building trust and dialog among different sectors is the IOM Food Forum, where trust is built by sharing different perspectives and through maintaining a continued dialog.
- **Provide decision makers with recommendations based on science.** An authoritative Mexican institution could make recommendations on nutritional issues as a basis for government policy making in a manner similar to the IOM process that is based on the best available science.
- **Developing prevention strategies.** All sectors in Mexico have the opportunity and responsibility to develop strategies based on the best available science and also drawing from the IOM report to adapt the recommendations to the Mexican context when appropriate.

BOX S-3 U.S.–Mexico Joint Obesity Prevention Task Force

Participants in Working Group III listed several elements for a U.S.–Mexico Obesity Prevention Task Force and include the following:

- **Advocacy.** Academia, industry, and the health sector need to communicate messages about the economic and health impact of obesity to the general public, government, and funding institutions.
- **Funding.** There are funding opportunities on both sides of the border, and collaboration will help in identifying potentially beneficial resources.
- **Training of labor force.** The creation of solutions to respond to malnutrition and obesity requires the Mexican labor force to be trained with new skills. Healthcare providers in the United States need to be trained in Mexican culture so they are able to give Mexican–American guidance on health and weight management.
- **Scientific evidence.** The scientific evidence for risk factors associated with obesity needs to continue to be gathered and shared.
- **Program evaluation.** There would be mutual benefits from sharing the information gathered from evaluating the efficacy of programs and interventions.
- **Consistency in programs and messages.** As the United States and Mexico increase their cultural and commercial exchanges, actions in both countries need to occur in parallel and in a coordinated fashion to avoid inconsistent and counterproductive policies, guidances, and educational programs.

1

Overview

The Institute of Medicine (IOM) in the United States and the National Institute of Public Health (Instituto Nacional de Salud Pública, INSP) in Mexico organized and co-sponsored a two-day workshop at INSP's headquarters in Cuernavaca, Morelos, Mexico with support from Kaiser Permanente (see agenda in Appendix A). The primary objective of the workshop was to explore the potential for a binational obesity prevention strategy for Mexican and Mexican–American (U.S. children of Mexican heritage) children and youth; the strategy should consider the perspectives, visions, and experiences of various stakeholders—governments, research institutions, industry, nongovernmental organizations, and communities. Additional workshop objectives included assessing similarities and differences in obesity prevention for Mexican and Mexican–American children, sharing policy and program experiences so that the options to prevent the childhood obesity epidemic are selected, and identifying data and information gaps. This summary highlights discussion items focusing particularly on the nature of childhood obesity, its magnitude and distribution, and current and future policies and programs (especially on the potential of binational collaborative responses); participants also discussed lessons learned from describing current interventions. Two background papers—"Preventing Obesity in Mexican Children and Adolescents" and "Preventing Obesity in Mexican–American Children and Adolescents"—describe the perspective of the obesity problem in Mexican–American and Mexican children and youth and were the basis for much of the workshop discussions (see Appendixes B and C, respectively).

The following are highlights from welcoming remarks by Juan Rivera (INSP), Mauricio Hernández (INSP), Jaime Sepúlveda (Ministry of Health), and Reynaldo Martorell (Emory University). As Rivera emphasized, the already-high prevalence of obesity in children on both sides of the U.S.–Mexico border has been increasing. The devastating effects of obesity on health threaten to increase the burden of health services and affect not only the health but also the productivity of the population. For this reason obesity is undoubtedly one of the major problems of public health in Mexico as well as in the United States.

Sepúlveda welcomed members of the audience and reflected on the decades of productive collaborations between INSP and a number of U.S. institutions—the CDC (Centers for Disease Control and Prevention), Emory University, and IOM—that provide the foundation for opportunities like this workshop. He applauded the participation of expert leaders from government (including executive and legislative councils), the private sector, the community, and the academic sector (see list of participants in Appendix D). Hernández and Martorell welcomed the audience on behalf of INSP and IOM, respectively, and described the organizations' roles as public health institutions. Hernández explained that INSP's mission is to contribute to social equity through research in public health, innovation of health systems, and the formation of highly qualified experts in Mexico. Reynaldo Martorell, a member of IOM's Food and Nutrition Board, described IOM as a private, nonprofit organization that is part of the National Academies and serves as an advisor to the United States to improve health. As an independent scientific advisor, the organization provides unbiased, evidence-based advice to many sectors including policy makers, health professionals, industry, and the public.

Origins and Evolution

Martorell, who served as chair of the planning committee, described the program and its origins. He explained the circumstances that led to this workshop:

- Childhood obesity is a global health problem. Health authorities in Mexico and the United States have recognized obesity as an important public health problem and as a result have initiated the development and, in some cases, the implementation of preventative and control policies and programs.
- Among the U.S. population, Mexican Americans, particularly Mexican–American women, are among the most affected by this epidemic.
- The United States and Mexico share many similarities and are integrated in many respects—language, culture, food, media, and economy—

due in part to the continuous, increasing exchange of people and product trading.

IOM and INSP public health experts considered these factors and initiated a dialog. It became clear that the scientific community, the healthcare community, and decision makers have the responsibility of joining efforts to prevent childhood obesity and to explore collaboration in research, prevention programs, and policies. Accordingly, leaders on both sides of the border agreed that the time was right to organize a workshop for initiating dialogue among all key players.

The workshop's general objectives were to share experiences and to consider the development of a binational agenda for preventing obesity in Mexican and Mexican–American children. The workshop planning committee [Reynaldo Martorell (*Chair*), Jeffrey Koplan, and Juan Rivera (with the assistance of IOM staff Maria Oria, Vivica Kraak, and Linda Meyers)] developed the workshop program.

Workshop Program

Appendix A is the complete workshop agenda. After the welcoming remarks, Jeffrey Koplan, chair of the Committee on Prevention of Obesity in Children and Youth, summarized highlights from the IOM report *Preventing Childhood Obesity: Health in the Balance* (2005), which was published at the request of the U.S. Congress and recommends an action plan for addressing childhood obesity in the United States. His presentation was followed by the summaries of the two background papers (presented by the authors) on prevention of obesity of Mexican and Mexican–American children and youth.

The remainder of the workshop program focused on fostering dialogue among all participants through small working groups, panels, or plenary sessions. Three working groups—whose participants were chosen for their expertise, country of origin, and personal interests—compared the status of the obesity epidemic in the United States and Mexico and explored questions on the prevalence, associated causes, and intervention programs; identified and discussed research gaps; and developed potential strategies and specific activities appropriate and beneficial for a U.S.–Mexico program (Martorell emphasized that this deliberation would be a central focus of the workshop). The findings from the working groups are included in this summary.

Representatives from various public and private sectors shared U.S. and Mexican perspectives on the roles of the private and public sectors in preventing childhood obesity; these perspectives are included in the section of this summary on "Solutions to Prevent Obesity in Children and Youth of

Mexican Origin." Finally, the workshop concluded with remarks from Reynaldo Martorell, Jeffrey Koplan, Juan Rivera, Jaime Sepúlveda, and Julio Frenk. Verbatim remarks from Jaime Sepúlveda and Julio Frenk (Ministry of Health) are included in the "Final Remarks" section of this summary. This summary should not be perceived as a series of recommendations reached by consensus but rather as a recapitulation of the discussions of working groups and individual participants.

For consistency, the definitions of obese and at-risk for obesity in this report were borrowed from those in the IOM report *Preventing Childhood Obesity: Health in the Balance* (2005). Hence, *obese children or youth* refers to those with age- and gender-specific BMI that is equal to or greater than the 95th percentile of the CDC body mass index (BMI)[1] charts. The IOM report defines *children and youth at-risk for obesity* as those with BMI-for-age 85th percentile to less than 95th percentile. On some occasions, participants also use the terms *overweight children* and *at-risk for overweight children.*

This summary and the appendixes will be available in Spanish and English.

REFERENCE

IOM (Institute of Medicine). 2005. *Preventing Childhood Obesity: Health in the Balance.* Washington, DC: The National Academies Press.

[1]Body mass index (BMI) is an indirect measure of body fat calculated as the ratio of a person's body weight in kilograms to the square of a person's height in meters. In children and youth, BMI is based on growth charts for age and gender and is referred to as BMI-for-age, which is used to assess underweight, overweight, and risk for overweight.

BMI (kg/m^2) = weight (kilograms) ÷ height $(meters)^2$

BMI (lb/in^2) = weight (pounds) ÷ height $(inches)^2 \times 703$

2

Background

HEALTH IN THE BALANCE: RECOMMENDATIONS FOR THE U.S. POPULATION

The childhood obesity epidemic was recognized in the United States as well as in other places around the world; it is an alarming trend in children of all ages. Figure 2-1 shows that the percentages of obese children have doubled in the early teen years and tripled for children in the 6–11 years of age range. The epidemic affects millions of children in the United States, and its persistence is clear. The reasons for the concern over the obesity prevalence increase stems largely from its very serious comorbidities (see Box 2-1), including a predisposition toward diabetes—a new form of the disease that formerly occurred only in adults. The onset of child diabetes used to be a more genetically determined disease, however, there now is a need to shift strategies because of the change in disease patterns.

Jeffrey Koplan, chair of the Committee on Prevention of Obesity in Children and Youth, summarized highlights from the IOM report *Preventing Childhood Obesity: Health in the Balance* (2005). The report was published after two years of deliberations by the committee and support from the CDC, the National Institutes of Health, the Office of Disease Prevention and Health Promotion of the Department of Health and Human Services, and the Robert Wood Johnson Foundation. The study was a collaboration between the IOM's Food and Nutrition Board and the Board on Population Health and Public Health Practice. The final report was produced by a diverse committee of 19 people and in accordance with IOM procedures.

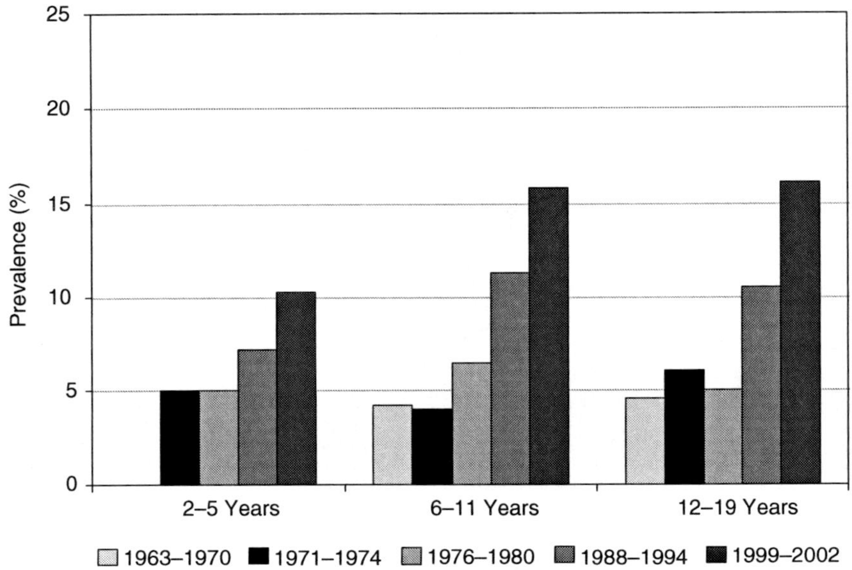

FIGURE 2-1 Childhood obesity prevalence, 1963–2002.
SOURCE: Hedley et al. (2004).

BOX 2-1 Implications for Children and Society: Physical, Social, and Emotional Health Consequences of Obesity

Physical Health
Glucose intolerance
Insulin resistance
Type 2 diabetes
Hypertension
Dyslipidemia
Hepatic Steatosis
Cholelithiasis
Sleep apnea
Orthopedic problems

Emotional Health
Low self-esteem
Negative body image
Depression

Social Health
Stigma
Negative stereotyping
Discrimination
Teasing and bullying

SOURCE: IOM (2005).

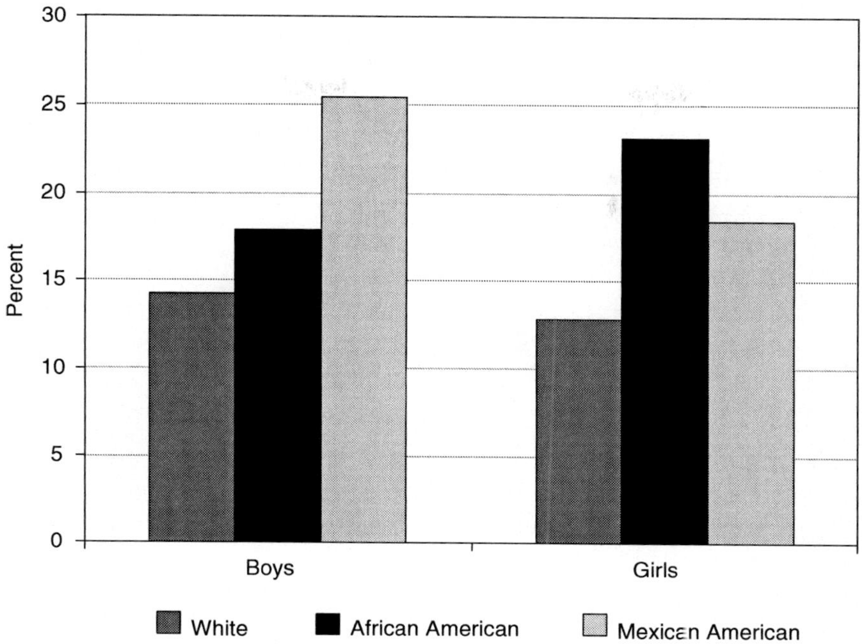

FIGURE 2-2 Childhood obesity prevalence in children 6–19 years old in 1999–2002.
SOURCE: Hedley et al. (2004).

In their search for interventions to prevent obesity, committee members and members of the public offered many single solutions—for example, eliminating vending machines from schools, increasing physical activity levels, and eliminating sweetened carbonated beverages or fast foods. However, although these elements might be contributory and important in childhood obesity prevention, the committee shared the view that a comprehensive study of the entire environment and all the sub-populations in the United States would be important in recognizing and understanding the elements' interrelations and how they impacted childhood obesity. To show the severity of the problem, Koplan presented Figure 2-2 with trend data for obesity prevalence from 1963 to 2002 among some U.S. ethnic populations.

The committee decided early in the study that although more research is needed before there is unequivocal scientific evidence to take definitive, specific actions, waiting for the evidence before taking action would be irresponsible. Because the problem is so urgent and widespread, the committee recommended that actions be taken based on the best available evidence, rather than waiting for the best possible evidence. The committee was careful, though, to emphasize the need for further evaluation and measurement of the recommended actions since many have not been validated. This need to measure the effectiveness of the applied interventions within and across different sectors is the focus of an ongoing IOM study on the progress in preventing childhood obesity (IOM, 2007).The study emphasizes the importance of evaluating programs and interventions in government, industry, schools, communities, and at home.

The committee concluded that childhood obesity is a serious nationwide health problem with multi-factorial causes requiring a population-based prevention approach and a comprehensive response. The committee also concluded that it is important to maintain energy balance for children and youth through the promotion of healthy eating behaviors and regular physical activity. Achieving energy balance is a process that relies on equalizing calories consumed versus calories expended. The goal, therefore, is to create energy balance in which physical activity and a healthful diet merge to improve the long-term health of future adults. Since preventing childhood obesity is a collective responsibility, this goal will be realized only by actively engaging many players and sectors, including parents, schools, governments, the food and beverage industry, the advertising industry, the physical activity industry, community groups, volunteer groups, and professional organizations such as medical and health groups (see Box 2-2). During the workshop, Koplan suggested that this concept of collective responsibility also might apply to Mexico.

BOX 2-2 Key Stakeholders Involved in *Preventing Childhood Obesity*

- Families,
- Schools,
- Communities,
- Healthcare groups,
- Industry,
- Media, and
- Government.

SOURCE: IOM (2005).

Unfortunately, society is typically crisis-driven; that is, only when faced with an acute public health issue does society respond with sufficient leadership and resources to mitigate it. Childhood obesity prevention is a long-term goal, and just as it took years for obesity to develop into an epidemic, the timeframe to begin reversing the problem might take years of coordinated multidisciplinary interventions. Because the rise in obesity prevalence has occurred over a long period of time and because it brings a complicated picture of contributors and solutions, the response has been inadequate.

Koplan emphasized that it is important not to undermine the interesting activities evolving in the communities, schools and school systems, and YMCAs, activities helping to change social norms (e.g., driving instead of walking, paying less money but receiving larger food servings, and using the elevator instead of the stairs) and encourage a reversal of the obesity problem. Also, Koplan noted that societal norm changes in countries such as Australia or Western Europe could serve as positive models for change. Although changing societal norms may seem like an insurmountable task, there are examples of successful health programs that have effected changes in social norms in the United States, for example, highway safety, tobacco control, and attitudes toward drinking and driving.

The IOM report's action plan includes a series of specific recommendations. For example, when targeting families and home life, the action plan recommends breastfeeding over other means, and for governments it recommends ensuring that all school meals meet the Dietary Guidelines for Americans. The report engages the whole society, including parents and healthcare providers, as part of the solution. There is undoubtedly an element of individual responsibility associated with making food choices; however, children cannot differentiate between health messages and pure product marketing, so individual responsibility becomes a less significant factor in the case of childhood obesity. Koplan stated that even though individuals need to make the right choices, society (e.g., industry, schools, government, and parents) needs to help.

OBESITY IN CHILDREN AND YOUTH OF MEXICAN ORIGIN: A SILENT BUT ALARMING EPIDEMIC

As mentioned by Rivera, obesity is undoubtedly one of the major public health problems in Mexico, and the devastating effects of obesity on health threaten to raise the burden of health services and affect not only the health but also the productivity of the population.

Sepúlveda highlighted indicators of the obesity epidemic in Mexico. He pointed out that according to the Organization of American States (http://www.oas.org), among its 30-country membership, Mexico sits in second place as far as having the highest rates of prevalence for obesity and risk for obesity. In Mexico, an anthropometric review of survey household data revealed that almost 29 percent of the country's preschool children are obese or at-risk of becoming obese (based on the U.S. reference population and definitions). In Mexican schools, one of every five children is obese. In the adult population, two-thirds of all men and women have tendencies toward obesity or are obese, and one of every five Mexicans is obese. Moreover, according to the last National Health Survey (Olaiz et al., 2003) 8 percent of the Mexican population is diabetic, and 30 percent of Mexican adults have hypertension. The metabolic syndrome that accompanies obesity—which includes hypertension, hypercholesterolemia, and cardiovascular disease—is burdening Mexican public health, to a magnitude not yet realized. To add to the complexity of the obesity epidemic, there is still a serious problem of malnutrition and micronutrients deficiency in Mexico.

Despite the alarming trends and existence of survey systems (e.g., the National Health and Nutritional Surveys) and national programs (e.g., Progresa and Oportunidades), Sepúlveda acknowledged these findings have not yet been translated into government decisions and public policies. Mexican authorities and society in general have not initiated preventative strategies.

The information in this section summarizes presentations by the authors of the two background papers—"Preventing Obesity in Mexican Children and Adolescents" and "Preventing Obesity in Mexican–American Children and Adolescents." For more details on the data available on obesity prevalence among Mexican and Mexican–American children and youth see Appendixes B and C, respectively.

Fernando Mendoza, Stanford University School of Medicine, introduced the workshop audience to the cultural factors that define the Latino family and to the acculturation process they experience as they integrate into U.S. society. These factors are key to understanding the causes of obesity and proposing solutions. For example, a traditional Latino family holds strong Mexican cultural and religious traditions; when the acculturation process begins their traditional lifestyles change. The nature of these changes as they relate to factors that contribute to obesity is not fully understood, but it appears that U.S. social norms with respect to diet and exercise are adopted by Mexican Americans as they acculturate into mainstream society. Latinos, the largest minority population in the United States, represent 14 percent of the U.S. population and are predicted to represent about 25 percent by 2030 (NRC, 2006). From that Latino population, almost two-thirds are Mexican American, so Mexican Americans are the most prominent Latino group in the United States (see Figure 2-3). Because of the continued influx of Mexicans and other Latinos into the United States, there is a range of acculturation levels among them. Figure 2-4 shows the dramatic changes in the U.S. population throughout the century due to immigration

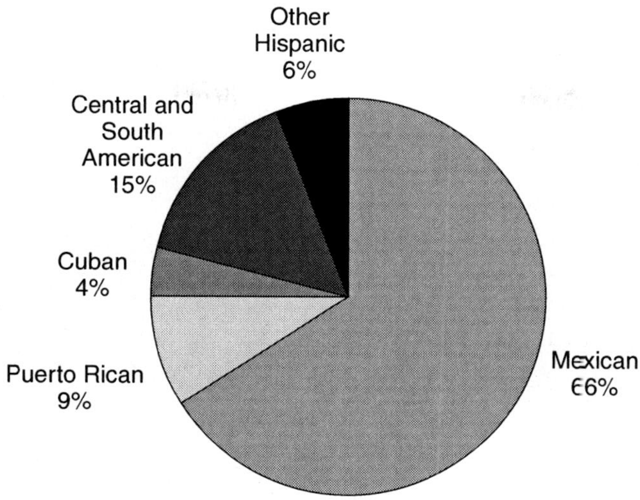

FIGURE 2-3 Percent distribution of Hispanics by type in the United States.
SOURCE: Current Population Survey, March, 2000, PGP-4.

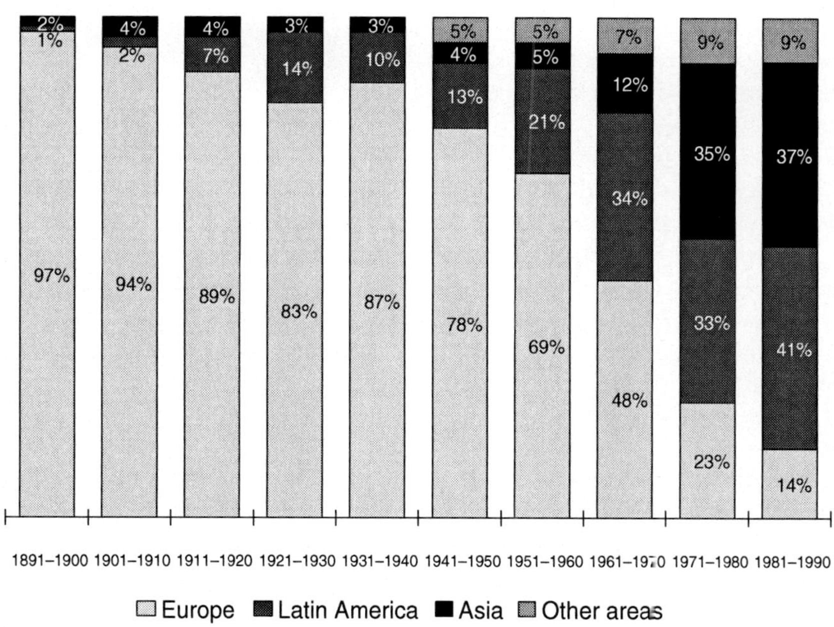

FIGURE 2-4 Documented immigration by area of origin.
SOURCE: Personal communication, Jorge Del Pinal (1995).

from Europe, Latin America (principally Mexico), and Asia. Vivid examples of states where the majority of the population is no longer white but people of color (primarily Latinos) include New Mexico, Texas, California, and Arizona. Approximately one third of California's population is Latino (primarily Mexican American); half of the babies born in California are either Mexican Americans or of other Latino heritage. This increase in the Latino population has spurred a great interest among policy makers and public-life leaders.

Mendoza pointed to the fact that for many years the health and social concerns among Mexicans in the United States went unnoticed because the Mexican population was not large enough to be considered for surveys. Today Mexican Americans have problems with obesity, homicide, poverty, and accidents. The third National Health and Nutrition Examination Survey (NHANES) (Burgos et al., 2005) shows that in the early 1990s 75 percent of the first generation of Mexican Americans was in poverty, two-thirds were uninsured, and approximately 80 percent possessed less than a ninth-grade education. The higher poverty rate of Mexican Americans compared with other non-Latino whites appears to continue into the second and even third generations. Thus, poverty is an issue both for Mexican and Mexican Americans, and as such its environmental correlates are important factors to examine in the evaluation of obesity among Mexican and Mexican Americans. Even though genetic factors might provide a predisposition to obesity, the environment is really what makes the biggest difference between being obese and non-obese and, in general, having good and poor health. The hope is that with the increase in the Mexican–American population greater attention will be given to this population, and public policy will address obesity and other health disparities affecting them. With new leaders such as Antonio Villaraigosa in public policy, the mayor in Los Angeles, the city with the largest population of Mexicans outside Mexico, positive changes may happen.

Robert Valdez, Univision Communication Corporation's "Salud es Vida: ¡Enterate!," added that a complex cultural transition process is happening not only in the United States but also in Mexico and is reflected in the differences between northern and southern Mexico that developed over the last several years. In addition, there is a third emergent culture along the U.S.–Mexican border where the cities on both sides are becoming more similar. Understanding the basic principles; causes; and social, psychological, and economic consequences of this cultural adaptation process will allow researchers and players in other sectors to better understand and prevent the obesity problem.

For the purposes of this workshop and background papers, children at-risk for obesity were defined as those with a BMI in the 85–95th percentile, and obese children were defined as those with a BMI in percentiles higher

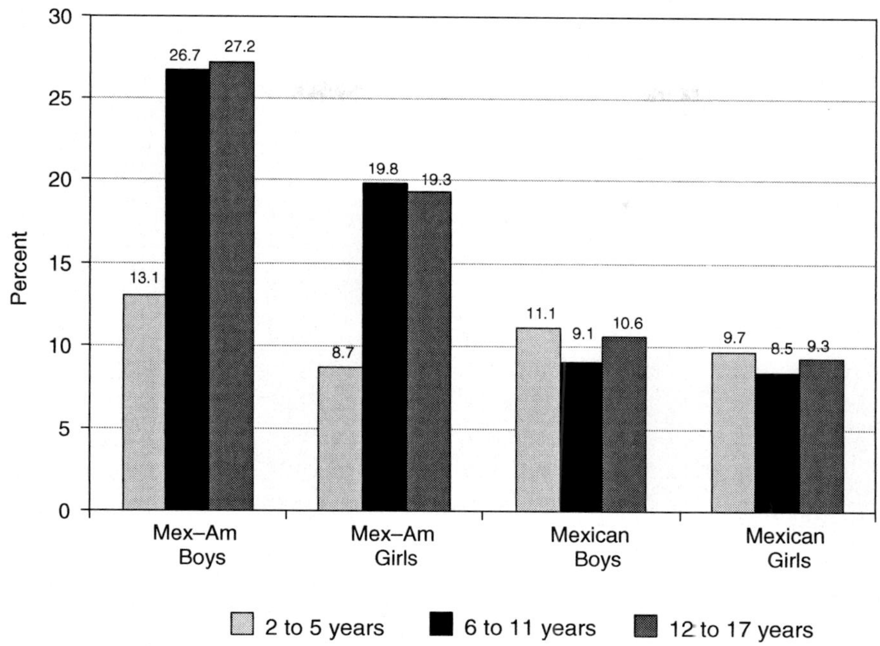

FIGURE 2-5 Obesity prevalence in Mexican–American and Mexican Children, 1999–2000.
SOURCE: Rivera et al. (2002) and del Rio-Navarro et al. (2004).

than the 95th. BMI, rather than waist circumference, was used as an obesity indicator because not only is it currently the parameter most commonly used but also it is standardized and easy to measure. Whether measured by BMI or waist circumference, the obesity issue in the United States is most urgent among the Mexican–American community (see Figure 2-5). In fact, the summary of epidemiological data in Appendix C indicates that among various ethnic groups (i.e., White, African American, and Mexican American), Mexican Americans show the highest obesity prevalence in both the 2–5- and 6–11-year-old boys. A similar conclusion is drawn from obesity prevalence data in girls. Clearly, preventing obesity in Mexican–American children presents an important public health challenge; the problem is also severe among other ethnic groups.

Comparing only the U.S. and Mexican–American populations in Figure 2-5, Mexican–American boys and girls are more obese in the older-age groups and somewhat more obese in the younger-age groups. The problem affects the entire U.S. population, with an increase in obesity in boys from 14 percent to 18 percent, a 30 percent increase from the 1980s to the 1990s.

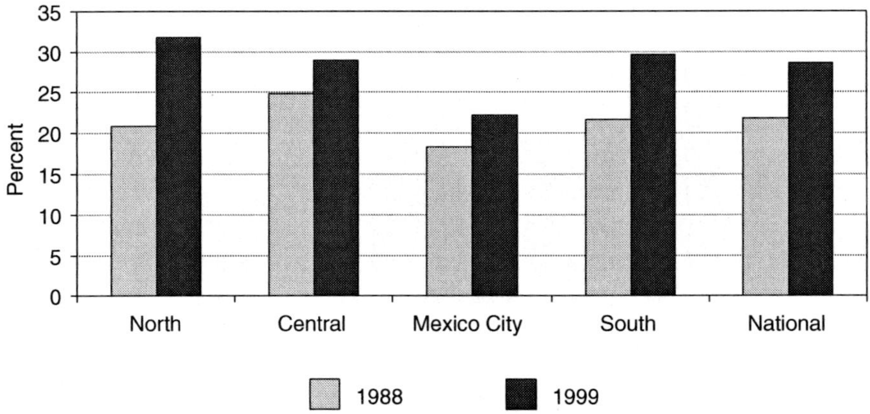

FIGURE 2-6 Prevalence of obesity or at risk for obesity by region and year of survey (children ages 2–4 years).
SOURCE: Rivera et al. (2001).

Mendoza reminded the audience that the obesity epidemic for Mexican Americans is nothing new and was recognized from all the NHANES surveys; for the first time, however, it has been recognized publicly not only as a national issue but also as an issue that greatly affects Mexican Americans.

Ruy López, INSP, presented a summary of the data on obesity prevalence in Mexico, where the nature of the obesity epidemic in children 2 to 4 years of age can be appreciated from the National Nutrition Surveys conducted in 1988 and 1999 (see Appendix B and Figure 2-6). Although it can be argued that the parameters used here and in Appendix B might not constitute ideal indicators of obesity or risk of obesity in the Mexican population because the reference is the U.S. population, the authors argued that those indicators should be used until a more appropriate reference population database is developed.

Martorell commented that the prevalence levels underestimate the obesity problem because of the reference curves used; he compared the reference curves to the World Health Organization's (WHO's) new growth curves for children under 5 years of age, based on studies done in Brazil, India, Ghana, Oman, Norway, and the United States with breastfed children of a high socioeconomic level. Martorell believes that these new curves should be used in the future because they reflect optimal growth as compared with the growth curves currently used (see also Appendix C). It is critical that the public be informed about the value of their use and that researchers coordinate and compare data across countries. Rivera suggested that data currently being collected on malnutrition, overweight issues, obesity, and risk of chronic disease from the third National Survey on Health and Nutrition could be analyzed using the WHO's new reference curves so that consensus on interpretation could be reached. Regardless, a preliminary assessment of the data indicates that several prevalences, including those for low weight for size, low size for age, and obesity, will increase.

Lopez noted that despite these questions a study by Villalpando (Villalpando el al., in press), which analyzed data from a national survey, demonstrates that children 10–19 years old showed a significantly higher glucose level before breakfast; higher levels of insulin, cholesterol, and triglycerides; and lower levels of high-density lipoproteins for obese or at-risk of obesity children than for normal weight children. These measurements are indicators of cardiovascular disease and demonstrate the severity of this problem in Mexico among obese or at-risk for obesity children.

Lopez concluded that it is clear from the survey data that the epidemic is real; however, information available at this time provides only suggestions for the possible risk factors associated with the epidemic. Based on the current epidemiological data, participants acknowledged that an obesity epidemic similar to the U.S. epidemic is also occurring in Mexico. Despite the limited information on potential risk factors associated with childhood obesity in Mexico, participants emphasized the urgency for key players to initiate preventative interventions for reversing the epidemic.

RISK FACTORS ASSOCIATED WITH CHILDHOOD OBESITY

This section summarizes the limited data on potential risk factors associated with childhood obesity in children and youth of Mexican heritage. For a more detailed description see Appendixes B and C. A discussion of the factors associated with this growing epidemic shows few controversies: authors of both background papers concluded that the lack of energy balance is the fundamental issue underlying the epidemic. However, when attempting to understand all the interrelated factors that make up the concept of energy balance they agreed that the picture is less clear. Intuitively, dietary factors and physical activity are the key factors but what are the environmental, genetic, physiological, or cultural factors that contribute to an energy balance? Lopez used Figure 2-7 (adapted from the 2005 IOM report *Preventing Childhood Obesity: Health in the Balance*) to represent an ecologic model that embraces interrelated factors affecting obesity.

Data for children 2–4 years old, the only age group for which data on trends exist in Mexico, suggest a similar increase in the prevalence of obesity as that seen in the United States (see Figure 2-6). Moreover, this figure shows that the prevalence of obesity is evident in all regions of the country. Lopez discussed the influence of socioeconomic status; in general, the preva-

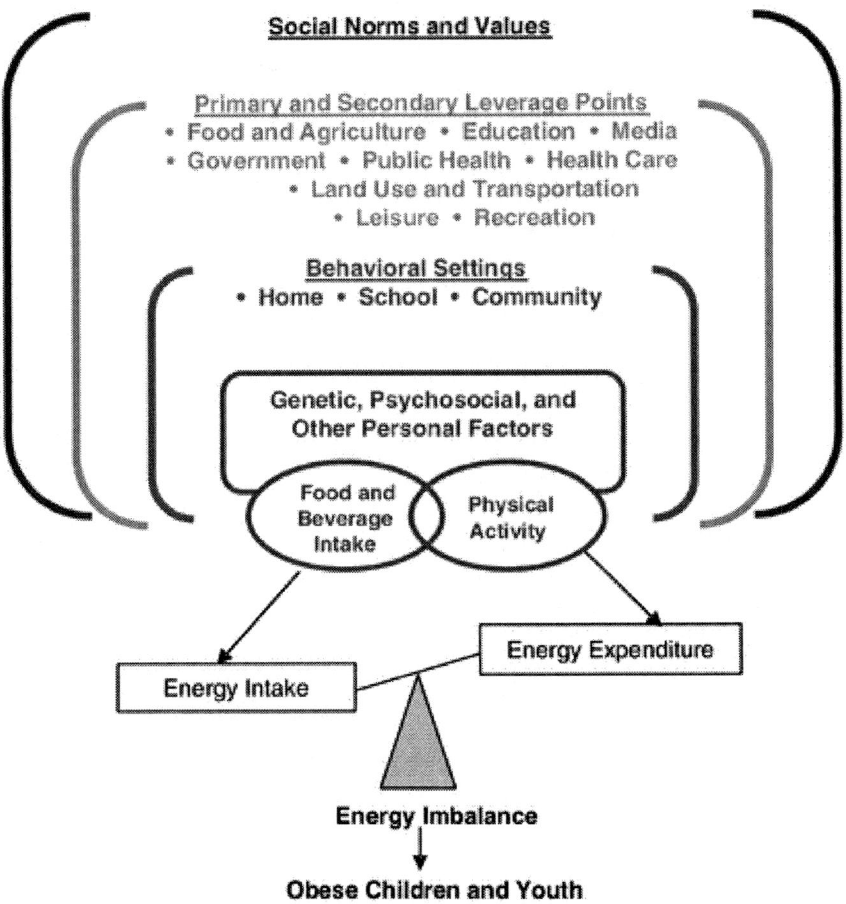

FIGURE 2-7 Factors influencing childhood obesity: ecological model.
SOURCE: IOM (2005).

lence of obesity in children increases as the socioeconomic level of the family increases. However, this is not the case in adults, where in the last two surveys associations among socioeconomic levels and obesity are the reverse. That is, the higher socioeconomic level of the family is associated with a lower prevalence of obesity. During the discussion, Rivera commented that the positive relationship between obesity and socioeconomic level in children implies that any program that improves wages in the population might also result in increases in the prevalence of childhood obesity.

In this sense he recommends that in programs like Mexico's Oportunidades, for example, improvements in income should happen in parallel with interventions to prevent obesity. The association between obesity and socioeconomic level seems to be different in the United States, where, in general, the more deprived sectors of society appear to have children with the highest rate of obesity (this association seems also to be the case for Mexican Americans). According to Rivera, an association between socioeconomic status and obesity similar to Mexico's also has been seen in Brazil; one explanation could be that this obesity trend is related to industrial development.

Several Mexican participants highlighted one factor that distinctly sets apart the obesity epidemic in Mexico, that is, the coexistence of obesity and malnutrition, sometimes within the same family. This dual burden of disease should be considered when identifying solutions, especially when the prevalence of malnutrition in Mexico is higher than in other Latin American countries. Wasting rate, a parameter that measures malnutrition in terms of weight for age, has decreased but low size for age continues to exist in Mexico and is associated with low socioeconomic status. Micronutrient deficiencies, including anemia in obese children, is also observed in Mexican populations.

The following sections underscore information on various factors, their interrelations, and their potential association with the obesity epidemic. Also, differences and similarities highlighted among the Mexican–American and Mexican populations are presented.

Diet-Related Factors

Frederick Trowbridge, Trowbridge and Associates, Inc., addressed the importance of psychosocial factors contributing to the high prevalence of obesity. He noted that these factors affect dietary habits and physical activity participation among Mexican immigrants as they integrate into U.S. culture. For example, U.S.-born Hispanics and long-term immigrants are much more likely to be obese than their foreign-born counterparts. U.S.-born Hispanics eat more fat and less fiber, as reported in dietary studies. Adolescents from more acculturated families eat more fat, protein, and calories. These findings point to changing dietary habits favoring obesity-prone diets. These changes in dietary habits also might originate from poverty and associated inaccessibility to affordable healthy foods.

Lopez described a different kind of nutritional transition occurring on the other side of the border, the one experienced by Mexicans in both urban and rural environments. Data from the 1988 and 1999 National Nutritional surveys (Barquera et al., in press) show an increase in fat intake and a decrease in carbohydrates intake. Income and Spending National Surveys report that spending for carbonated beverages, sodas, and refined carbohy-

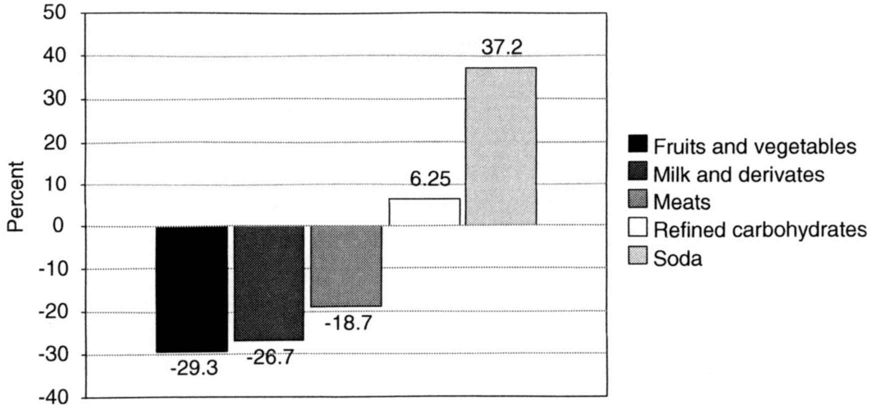

FIGURE 2-8 Changes in mean food purchases in 1996 (relative to 1994) by food group.
SOURCE: Rivera et al. (2004).

drates increased from 1994 to 1996; in contrast, spending for fruits and vegetables decreased, possibly because of high prices (see Figure 2-8). Additionally, data show that 60 percent of school children consume less than 100 grams of fruits and that only 8 percent of the school population follows the recommendation of five fruits or vegetables a day. Other food consumption data show that almost 40 percent of preschool-age children's energy comes from processed food; this appears to happen not only in urban areas but also in the rural environment.

Rivera and colleagues have collected research data that provides invaluable information about the situation in the school environment. The data suggest that childhood obesity is favored by a lack of water in schools (i.e., children substitute carbonated, high-calorie drinks for water), a lack of regulations or guidances appropriate for school food choices, and greater access to high-energy food than to nutritious food such as fruit.

Lopez stressed that although the evidence supporting the hypothesis that these foods contribute to obesity is unclear, there is enough information to believe that the transition in dietary habits might be contributing to obesity in the Mexican population. Concomitant with this dietary transition period, the fast food industry has grown, and street food in Mexico is being made with less healthy options such as cheaper, less healthy cooking oils.

Physical Activity-Related Factors

Trowbridge summarized the data regarding physical activity among Mexican Americans (see Appendix B). A literature review on physical activity revealed that free time physical activity self-reported by 9–13-year-old children and teenagers is similar in all the ethnic groups, but White, Non-Hispanics report much more participation in organized physical activity than African Americans or Hispanics; this finding may be related to unique barriers such as availability and expense to join an organized activity (i.e., entrance fees are required to join leagues), lack of transportation, availability of organized programs, and personal safety in the Mexican–American population as reported in the surveys.

Lopez presented Figure 2-9 to illustrate the results of a study by Bernardo Hernández in Mexico City that examined levels of physical activities in children 9–16 years old by income level. Regardless of the income level, the time spent viewing television and other videos is higher than the time spent on physical activity. The data from Mexico City showed that children who watch television for more than three hours daily have a 1.69-times higher risk of being obese than those who watch just one hour. (The

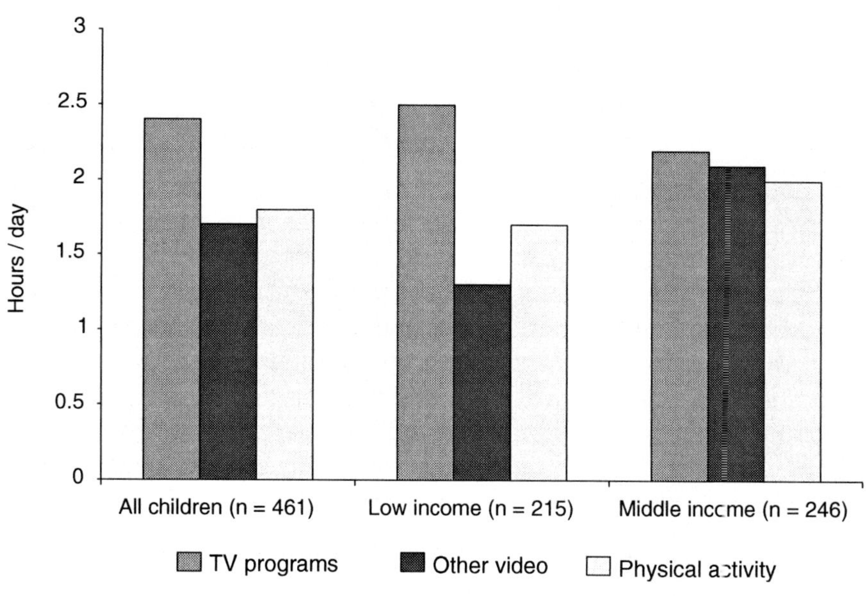

FIGURE 2-9 Levels of physical activity or inactivity. Mean time dedicated to video viewing and physical activity in children 9–16 years old in Mexico City.
SOURCE: Hernández et al. (1999).

recommendation by international experts is for children to engage in no more than two hours of screen viewing per day). Although there are no published national data on physical activity or its association with obesity, similar associations as in Mexico City have been found in other Mexican urban settings. Although no related survey data were found, personal safety could be an important barrier to Mexican children and youth engaging in physical activity, just as it is a barrier for the U.S. Hispanic population. In addition, a worrisome fact is that the school policies regarding physical activity are generally not followed, and 30 percent of the children do not enjoy physical activity at school, as observed in a small sample where physical activity constituted an average of only 10 minutes per day. In addition, extracurricular programs, which could add some physical exercise to children's daily activities, are very difficult to implement in Mexico.

Culture-Related Factors

As mentioned previously, sociopsychological and cultural factors play an important role in defining diet and physical activity habits of a population. Among them, culturally-based perceptions of body weight cannot be overlooked; for example, Trowbridge said that Hispanic mothers might be more likely to equate plumpness with healthy weight. Also, the strength of the idea of family is very powerful in Hispanic families and may have some unintended consequences on attitudes toward physical activity. For example, the CDC Youth Media Campaign Longitudinal Survey found that Hispanic youth were taught to put family needs above their own needs and that physical activity for their own benefit may be discouraged (see also Appendixes B and C and IOM, 2006). The lack of health insurance and access to healthcare might also constitute barriers to obesity prevention.

Several social and family factors seem to be unique in affecting Mexican dietary habits and some may remain as part of the Mexican heritage of the Mexican–American community in the United States. For instance, similar to the Mexican–American community, Lopez noted that although there is no scientific basis to confirm the idea that "chubby children are healthy children," it is very much engrained in low-income populations. Also, enjoying comforts and appliances such as television provides a certain desirable social status. The data about television access and Internet usage (see Appendix B) point to a higher use by children and youth over time, which could be seen as an opportunity (e.g., to communicate messages about health via television and the Internet) as well as a threat (e.g., supports the evidence of increased physical inactivity) for Mexican children. Nevertheless, increased car sales, television watching, and time spent on computers and the Internet suggest that Mexico is moving towards an obesogenic environment.

Regardless of the strength of the association between risk factors and the prevalence of obesity, the following are some critical elements that, according to Lopez, speak about the urgency of the matter:

- The prevalence of obesity among children is growing.
- The severity of the impact of obesity in both long-term health and economy could increase.
- Today's child and youth obesity epidemic will be observed in the future as children grow into adults.

This sense of urgency to take action against the obesity epidemic was transparent during the course of workshop discussions and was expressed in reference to both the United States and Mexico.

REFERENCES

Barquera S, Hotz C , Rivera J, Tolentino L, Espinoza J, Campos I, Shamah T. In press. Food consumption, food expenditure, anthropometric status, and nutrition-related diseases in Mexico. In: Kennedy et al., eds. *The Double-Burden of Diseases in Developing Countries.* Rome, Italy: Food and Agricultural Organization.

Burgos A, Schetzina K, Dixon B, Mendoza F. 2005. Importance of generational status in examining access to and utilization of health care services by Mexican American children. *Pediatrics* 115(3):322–330.

del Rio-Navarro BE, Velazquez-Monroy O, Sanchez-Castillo CP, Lara-Esqueda A, Berber A, Fanghanel G, Violante R, Tapia-Conyer R, James W. 2004. The high prevalence of overweight and obesity in Mexican children. *Obesity Research* 12:215–223.

Hedley AA, Ogden CL, Johnson CL, Carroll MD, Flegal KM. 2004. Prevalence of overweight and obesity among U.S. children, adolescents, and adults. *Journal of the American Medical Association* 91(23):2847–2850.

Hernández B, Gortmaker SL, Colditz GA, Peterson KE, Laird NM, Parra-Cabrera S. 1999. Association of obesity with physical activity, television programs and other forms of video viewing among children in Mexico City. *International Journal of Obesity* 23: 845–854.

IOM (Institute of Medicine). 2005. *Preventing Childhood Obesity: Health in the Balance.* Washington, DC: The National Academies Press.

IOM. 2007. *Progress in Preventing Childhood Obesity: How Do We Measure Up?* Washington, DC: The National Academies Press.

NRC (National Research Council). 2006. *Multiple Origins, Uncertain Destinies: Hispanics and the American Future.* Washington, DC: The National Academies Press.

Olaiz G, Rojas R, Barquera S, Shamah T, Aguilar C, Cravioto P, Lopez F, Hernandez M, Tapia R, Sepúlveda J. 2003. *Encuesta Nacional de Salud 2000, Tomo II.* La salud de los adultos. Cuernavaca, Morelos, México: Instituto Nacional de Salud Pública.

Rivera JA, Shamah-Levy T, Villalpando-Hernández S, González de Cossio T, Hernández-Prado B, Sepúlveda J. 2001. *Encuesta Nacional de Nutrición 1999.* Estado Nutricional en Niños y Mujeres en México, ed. Oropeza. Cuernavaca, Morelos, México: Instituto Nacional de Salud Pública.

Rivera JA, Barquera S, Campirano F, Campos I, Safdie M, Tovar V. 2002. Epidemiological and nutritional transition in Mexico: Rapid increase of non-communicable chronic diseases and obesity. *Public Health Nutrition* 5(1A):113–122.

Rivera JA, Barquera S, González-Cossio T, Olaiz G, Sepúlveda J. 2004. Nutrition transition in Mexico and in other Latin American countries. *Nutrition Reviews* 62(7):S149–S157.

Villalpando S, Carrión C, Barquera S. In press. The body mass index is associated with hyperglycemia and alterations of some components of the metabolic syndrome in Mexican adolescents aged 10–19 years. *Salud Pública de México*.

3

Opportunities and Challenges

OBESITY PREVENTION SOLUTIONS

From the available prevalence data on obesity and risk of obesity in children and youth (see Chapter 1), workshop participants agreed that there is enough evidence to prove that the epidemic is real and that society needs to move now from problem-oriented to solution-oriented research, which includes evaluations[1] of the interventions. Based on the risk factors already mentioned, a range of interventions in schools, media outlets, community venues, and healthcare facilities could be implemented, some of them jointly, to counterattack the obesity epidemic in Mexico and the United States.

A comparison between Mexican Americans and Mexicans highlights many commonalities; however, as pointed out by Jaime Sepúlveda, obvious differences in culture and social and political systems require careful analysis before recommendations for the United States are applied to Mexico. The U.S. experience and this joint workshop should serve as a springboard for Mexico to engage in a dialogue about strategies for the Mexican population. Sepúlveda concluded that the establishment of a Mexican Obesity Prevention Task Force that makes recommendations to the Mexican Ministries of Health and of Education is needed.

---

[1]Evaluation can be defined as a systematic assessment of the quality and effectiveness of an initiative, program, or policy and its effects, in order to produce information that can be used by those who have an interest in its improvement or effectiveness.

Workshop participants highlighted the following key issues as ones to consider in developing a framework for joint interventions:

- Interventions should focus on environmental changes that support individual behavior change (see discussion on the Berkley Media Series Group Report in Appendix B), and the strategy to mitigate the epidemic should be multilevel, multisectorial, and multidisciplinary.
- Larger populations could be served by paying attention to issues derived from scaling up the programs.
- Programs should be sustainable for the long term in terms of funding as well as feasibility.
- Collaboration with media is critical so that consistent information can reach children and youth through diverse venues.
- Developing appropriate (social and product) marketing campaigns for children and youth should be an integral intervention component.
- An ongoing scientific and programmatic exchange to share educational materials, research results, and evaluation of the interventions should be established.

During working group discussions it became apparent that the main determinants associated with obesity, highlighted in Figure 7 (Chapter 1), are similar in the two countries and are based on the one complex problem of balance between energy expenditure and energy intake. However, political, social, and economic differences do exist between the United States and Mexico, and researchers should consider those differences when sharing and implementing interventions based on each country's experiences. The following section highlights some of the barriers that might be encountered when implementing interventions.

Barriers and Challenges to Implementing Interventions

Most obesity prevention interventions present opportunities as well as challenges. The barriers that challenge our ability to combat the obesity epidemic can be divided into two categories: those related to specific interventions and those related to the social and political environment within which each population resides. For example, in the first category, using media to influence behaviors could be an effective intervention strategy to convey important messages; however, the use of media also can be counterproductive if used to promote unhealthy behaviors. Participants related that school- and community-based interventions also present challenges, such as finding additional resources and time dedicated to promoting obesity prevention. Time limitation is also one barrier often mentioned when considering healthcare interventions. With regard to the second category,

Mendoza (see Appendix B) expressed concerns over the lack of human resources and continuity in obesity research in the United States regarding Mexican–American children—leadership is needed urgently in coordinating all areas from interventions implementation to research and educational campaigns. Mendoza cited as an example of this disconnect the overwhelming amount of information in academic literature that rarely are synthesized to reach the local community, particularly disenfranchised communities (e.g., the poor or Hispanic). Also, generating leadership among the Mexican–American community would help increase the inclusion of Mexican Americans in the U.S. government agenda; this lack of leadership and inclusion of Mexican Americans on the agenda impedes progress in the obesity battle. Workshop participants generally agreed that a commitment to leadership needs to be made.

During the working groups and plenary discussions, barriers to alleviating the current epidemic that are unique to the social and political context of each country were highlighted and are listed below. Most of them apply to the United States as well as Mexico to some degree although participants discussed most of them in the Mexican context:

- In Mexico, the public lacks awareness of the obesity problem. Although this might not be the case at the government level, there is still not a sense of urgency among the public. Moreover, the problem is seen as complex and insurmountable. In the United States, the public, including the Mexican–American community, is much more aware of the problem. One limitation to action in the United States is that Mexican Americans are not being included in the government agenda setting and response.
- There is a lack of public trust in the government, industry, and academia.
- The number of food- and nutrition-related policies is scarce in Mexico, and those that exist are implemented and enforced inadequately.
- There is a lack of organizations that represent consumers; community empowerment and advocacy in Mexico are not common.
- In Mexico, there is an insufficient number of legislators who can translate and incorporate science into the legislative process and as a result government activities have centered on publishing findings instead of taking legislative actions.
- Nutritional transitions occurring at different times in the United States and Mexico might be related to differences in both nutritional problems and in socioeconomic distribution and to its relationship with obesity. For instance, in Mexico, stunting and micronutrient deficiencies continue to be of concern and coexist with obesity; while in Mexican–American communities micronutrient deficiencies also exist, the problem is less severe and obesity remains the larger problem. Also, there is an inverse relationship

between socioeconomic status and obesity in Mexican Americans and the opposite is true among Mexicans. These differences might actually provide an opportunity for implementing interventions as more is learned from the experience in both countries.

- Resources and instrumentalization to address health problems are inadequate.
- Gaps in scientific data are not always filled through strict scientific rigor.

Overcoming Barriers to Obesity Prevention

As a parallel strategy to the joint solutions described in a following section, Mexico needs a strategy of solutions particular to the Mexican context. Working Group III addressed this question and suggested that all sectors—academia, government, industry, nongovernmental organizations (NGOs), and other stakeholders—have the opportunity and responsibility to develop an obesity prevention strategy under a Mexican National Obesity Prevention Task Force. This strategy should take into account the urgency required by the continued rise in obesity and associated chronic diseases and the change in the Mexican government, and should be based on best available information. Martorell added that such a strategy could draw on the Institute of Medicine (IOM) report *Preventing Childhood Obesity* (IOM, 2005) but that it is equally important that the data generated in Mexico (e.g., from the National Health and Nutrition Survey) be used as a basis to support initiatives. Rivera reminded participants that there is a legal framework in Mexico based on a 2004 WHO (World Health Organization) General Assembly endorsement of the recommendations in the 2001 FAO (Food and Agriculture Organization) and WHO report *Diet, Physical Activity, and the Prevention of Obesity* (WHO, 2004). In this sense, Mexico has a commitment with WHO to develop a national strategy for obesity prevention, and therefore the efforts should continue. Rivera also suggested that the Mexican National Obesity Prevention Task Force and a U.S.–Mexico binational initiative could work synergistically.

The following are elements of the suggested Mexican National Obesity Prevention Task Force that reflect the discussions of Working Group III and further plenary discussions regarding activities where progress is needed in Mexico before (or concurrent to) the implementation of a binational agenda:

Increasing the awareness of the obesity problem. Public awareness in Mexico needs to be increased so that individuals are more receptive to preventative interventions. This could be done through a coordinated effort by the public health community, media, and government. Some participants believed that the collection of survey data with latest trends in obesity prevention (ENSANUT data), associated risks for other chronic diseases, and cost estimates of the obesity epidemic could be used as a basis to raise awareness among the healthcare, community and government sectors, and other decision makers.

Developing and implementing a national policy for obesity prevention. This national policy will have continuity regardless of changes in government. The school system in Mexico provides an extraordinary opportunity to implement changes that will affect a large part of the population (e.g., school foods or physical activity interventions). However, regulations or guidances will not help unless there are not financial and human resources to implement them. Also, in some cases, current regulations in Mexico are not always implemented or enforced. Regulations or guidances could follow those already implemented in other countries but considering also the Mexican political, social, and cultural context.

Participation of the community sector. Members of the community need to be educated, organized, and empowered to advocate to the government and funding institutions about health issues, and obesity in particular. Such an effort could assist the community sector in playing a pivotal role in advocacy and imparting positive changes. Community advocacy also provides an additional opportunity for collaboration among community, industry, and academic sectors. For example, the community could collaborate with industry on educating parents on obesity prevention.

Conducting a careful assessment of human resources. Mexico faces a dual burden of disease where micronutrient deficiency and obesity coexist. This new challenge calls for a careful assessment of human resources needs; for instance, there may be a need for experts in research evaluation, intervention efficacy, program management, and implementation. The United States can play an important role in providing assistance to build that capacity with appropriately designed training opportunities. The "Information and Research Gaps" section also provides some lead to specific research needs that might warrant innovative skills and training.

Building trust among various sectors. The group recognized that the only path toward long-term solutions for a multisectorial problem such as obesity must include collaboration and trust among sectors (e.g., industry, government, schools, and community). A mechanism by which such collaboration is initiated, Martorell noted, is the IOM's Food Forum, a successful model for building trust and dialog among different sectors. The Food Forum is composed of leaders from academia, government, industry, and consumers who meet regularly to discuss issues of common interest. When conducted under the umbrella of an independent institution like IOM, such a gathering fosters dialog and collaboration in a neutral and safe environment. Mutual trust is built by sharing different perspectives and through maintaining a dialog over time. Other specific interventions to build trust are described in the sections "Role of Families and Communities" and "Role of Industry." Strengthening the local public health capacity to collaborate with other sectors will help advance an obesity prevention agenda in multiple sectors.

Providing recommendations to decision makers based on scientifically-based research. It was the opinion of a number of participants that a study like the 2005 IOM report *Preventing Childhood Obesity: Health in the Balance* for the population of Mexican origin could be led by an authoritative Mexican institution that could make recommendations on nutrition and public health based on scientific evidence as well as highlight specific areas that warrant further research. For example, what are the risk factors (e.g., diets, socioeconomic status) in the different areas of Mexico that result in prevalence differences in the north and south? An effort could also be specifically directed to educating legislators about the obesity epidemic and potential solutions.

Developing prevention strategies. All sectors in Mexico have the opportunity and responsibility to develop strategies with a sense of urgency, taking into consideration the positive timing and based on the best available science and also drawing from the IOM report, that is, adapting the recommendations to the Mexican context when appropriate. In this respect, collaborations among all sectors are very important including the food industry but also other sectors such as food retailers and fast food chains.

Specific Interventions to Prevent Obesity in Children and Youth of Mexican Origin

Several participants maintained that the main premise for an obesity prevention strategy is that the causes of obesity follow on several levels an ecologic, causal model (see Figure 2-7) and, therefore, the strategy to mitigate the epidemic should be multilevel, multisectorial, and multidisciplinary. It also is important to recognize that interventions need to be based on the best available evidence and on data from solution-oriented research designs instead of problem-oriented research designs. Participants described solution-oriented research as research designs that lead directly to policy or practice changes that also include an evaluation component. Evaluating the efficacy of interventions and programs in preventing obesity is an important criterion to make decisions about which interventions merit further investment.

The following sections present a summary of the perspectives and experiences of U.S. and Mexican leaders from various sectors, including community, schools, industry, and government, plus other discussion items that were raised by workshop participants.

Role of Families and Communities

Carmen Rita Nevarez, Public Health Institute, provided a U.S. perspective on the distinct role that families and communities play in preventing childhood obesity. Changes in behavior do not happen easily or without the collaboration and agreement of families and communities. Nevarez addressed methods to engage the community in building healthier environments and emphasized ideas for necessary resources, tools, and skills.

Nevarez spoke from her broad experience in working with Californian communities, where there is an emphasis on environmental changes that encourage healthy choices by making them the easier alternatives. An example of the importance of community participation is demonstrated by the recent passage in California of two bills that create the strictest standard yet in the United States for food and beverages sold in public schools. The bills ban the sale of soda and other sweetened beverages in public schools starting in 2009. This outcome was possible because of community collaboration. Such collaboration included community members' participation in congressional committee hearings where young people, pediatricians, parents, and teachers expressed their health concerns and challenges in following a healthy lifestyle. The passage of those bills took a concerted effort to organize, educate, and bring the community to a level of trust and understanding so they could participate in the legislative process. It is clear that together with the public health authorities and experts, community leaders can transmit their ideas on necessary changes for communities to become healthy.

A current initiative in California is the Partners for Health project, sponsored by the California Endowment (a private California foundation that focuses on decreasing health and healthcare disparities). Under the Healthy Eating, Active Communities[2] initiative, five communities were selected to engage in school and community projects such as increasing the nontraditional exercises available at schools (e.g., walking to golf lessons) or evaluating cafeteria foods (e.g., increasing the fruits and vegetables options), turn-

---

[2]Healthy Eating, Active Communities (HEAC) is a four-year $26 million initiative of the California Endowment, the state's largest health philanthropy. HEAC's goal is to reduce disparities in diabetes and obesity by using community models and statewide policy advocacy to improve nutrition and physical activity environments in schools, neighborhoods, marketing and media, and by healthcare providers. Most of the places where HEAC is active are heavily populated by Mexican Americans. Improvements prompted by HEAC include enforcement of school nutrition and physical education standards, school wellness policies, health-conscious city planning, healthier options in vending machines in public venues, a teen recreation center, bike paths, farmers markets, and promotoras establishing a neighborhood playground (http://www.healthyeatingactivecommunities.org).

ing the teachers into the physical activity counselors, and assessing the health status of their environment.

The process by which a disenfranchised, poor, Latino community can engage in community initiatives, particularly related to health, involves gaining the trust of a *promotora*—a trained individual who communicates healthy messages and helps others learn to be advocates by teaching people about health and communication skills, especially on how to communicate with authorities. The role of the promotoras is key to building trust between community members and authorities and should be supplemented with regular meetings among community members and the city council or the local health department. Finally, and most importantly, youth should contribute (and be accepted for) their energy, ideas, and participation—they are invaluable resources to influence decision making and changes in the community.

As mentioned previously, many regulations, health policies, and initiatives on preventing obesity and other health problems originate from social, nongovernmental, or consumer organizations that are supported by the community. Mexican workshop participants reiterated that in Mexico there unfortunately is not a sector that supports and represents the interests of consumers; therefore, Mexico's efforts in developing an obesity prevention roadmap in which community engagement is a key factor are limited but should be pursued.

Role of Schools

Guillermo Ayala, Mexican Secretaria de Educación Pública (Ministry of Public Education), presented a Mexican perspective on how schools could contribute to the implementation of solutions for mitigating the obesity epidemic. In his view, schools play a role not only in nutrition education but also in the development of critical thinking skills (e.g., decision-making skills and those required to overcome social pressure).

Mexican schools follow the regulations published in the Federal Official Newspaper (Diario Oficial de la Federación) in 1882. The functions of the Social Participatory School Board (Consejo Escolar de Participación Social en las Escuelas) are described in the Guidelines for the Organization and Functioning of Elementary Schools and Adult Education (Lineamientos para la Organización y Funcionamiento de las Escuelas de Educación Básica, Inicial, Especial y para Adultos). The Board's members are the school principal, parents, representatives of their associations, teachers, and union representatives working in collaboration with interested members of the community. In this venue, Ayala said, the participation of the private sector (e.g., the food industry) would be beneficial.

Ayala presented data on the prevalence of obesity in schools—information that reiterates the urgency of the problem. An assessment of the school situation found that in 2004–2005, the prevalence of obesity among preschool children was only 2 percent and remained low in 2005–2006. However, in elementary schools, the prevalence of obesity in 2005–2006 was 24 percent—a worrisome increment given the detrimental consequences to health, according to Ayala.

In terms of physical activity, the General Board of Physical Education (Dirección General de Educación Física) developed a physical activity program in Mexico City schools that stimulates daily physical education before classes start and evaluates its efficiency. Unfortunately, as acknowledged by other participants, some past policies on physical education have led to a situation where some Mexican states provide insufficient levels of physical education. The national program of physical education for the whole country should be seen as an opportunity and should remain in place regardless of the changes in the government. Institutions like SEP (Secretaria de Educación Pública, Secretary of Public Education) and Instituto Nacional de la Salud Pública (INSP) as well as the healthcare sector in general would serve as advisors to the government in developing a national program.

Another intervention that is proving to be invaluable in schools is involving children in health programs. For example, the Interdisciplinary Committee on Diabetes, Obesity and Cardiovascular Diseases (Comité Interdiciplinario para la Diabetes, Obesidad y Enfermedades Cardiovasculares) has initiated a program that includes prediagnosis of obesity and realistic, practical objectives for decreasing obesity in schools. Ayala added that to guarantee progress, schools need to develop an integrated system—one that includes schools as well as physicians—around promoting and maintaining health needs. In that regard, researchers should find motivational factors for physicians so that the doctors monitor obesity in their routine check-ups. Changes toward a healthy lifestyle can be encouraged in many ways but the cooperation of physicians is key to initiating and continuing those changes. Diana Bonta, Kaiser Permanente, provided examples of viable, yet challenging, next steps to increase the healthcare sectors participation in preventing obesity like requiring body mass index (BMI) be part of the medical chart and training physicians to communicate about obesity.

In addition to interventions, there are systems research projects at the schools conducted primarily by INSP and the General Board of Epidemiology (Dirección General de Epidemiología) from the Ministry of Health. Information based on their research has led to the implementation of school interventions. For example, the General Board of Epidemiology (Dirección General de Epidemiología) from the Ministry of Health, is conducting a study on overweight and obesity control in the schools of Mexico City from a clinical perspective. Ayala expects that new recommendations for interventions will continue to be based on updated, improved surveys conducted in collaboration with the schools. In addition, the studies will undoubtedly result in a new research agenda for the 2006–2007 school cycle that will incorporate cross-sectional and longitudinal studies for collecting data on many aspects of changing behaviors. The school systems need clear, efficient recommendations for interventions. Collaboration with industry would be beneficial in the developing of such recommendations.

Ayala and others recognized that a more severe limitation to increasing the level of physical education classes in schools is the lack of economic resources to invest in physical activities, sports facilities, and didactic materials for the teachers. There are some programs for physical education, but they have been neither applied nor evaluated. There is a general sense that an additional limitation to intervention progress at the schools is the amount of bureaucracy. Russell Pate, University of South Carolina, added a general comment on other broader, intrinsic challenges related to sustaining an active life for the long term, that is the provision of experiences that not only provide enjoyment and a sense of competence as children but also later as adults. Although there is a lack of research data to support the long-term impact of exercising as a child, Pate asserted that it contributes to lifelong good habits resulting from increased confidence in an ability to be active and enjoyment in the activity. This is an area where the United States needs improvement, too, because as many as 40 percent of high school students report not being involved in interscholastic sports.

Although, some preventive actions are being implemented by improving nutrition and guaranteeing daily physical activity, educating children (as well as teachers and the general public) on obesity prevention through effective campaigns is critical. Ultimately, there is still not enough nutrition information in school programs.

Role of Industry

What actions can industry, restaurants, caterers, media, and advertising and marketing agencies take to continue to reverse and prevent the obesity epidemic in youth and children? Should the food industry produce healthier food or try to modify behavior in children and youth; should the industry take an active role in encouraging parents and community members to be role models? This section summarizes thoughts on these questions from a U.S. and Mexican perspective.

Food industry. Lance Friedman from Kraft Co. presented his perspective and a summary of activities initiated by Kraft Co. The following are key elements of Kraft's health and wellness strategy: healthier food is not only good for public health but also can be translated into company revenue; self-regulation of the food industry can be an effective way of providing healthy choices to the public; and given the complexity of the obesity problem, collaboration is the only real path to success in providing the public with appropriate information and healthy food choices, in marketing campaigns that foster behavioral changes, and in implementing other food industry interventions. He referred to *Preventing Childhood Obesity: Health in the Balance* (IOM, 2005) for a comprenhensive account of measures that could be taken by industry.

Two areas where Friedman envisions the role of industry are gaining the trust with stakeholders and the public and increasing the range of healthy products (e.g., Kraft's "better for you products"). To grow public trust in industry, an advisory board was established to develop program ideas in the following four areas: improving the overall nutrition profile of products, providing more and better consumer information, practicing responsible marketing to help children to make the right choices, and participating in advocacy and dialogue.

Among the many initiatives to include in the "better for you products" campaign, a critical one is to encourage consumption of healthier products through the development of specific logos identifying healthier products such as the "Sensible Solution" products, which meet nutrition standards like calorie, fat, sugar, and sodium reduction; an increase in beneficial nutrients (such as calcium, whole grain, fiber, and protein); or inclusion of functional benefits (such as heart health). A parallel program—"Elección equilibrada"—has been implemented in Mexico. In terms of marketing, the U.S. and European agencies continue to deliberate on appropriate food marketing policies for children.

Extending healthy lifestyle programs beyond food products into community programs (e.g., "Salsa Sabor y Salud" and "Alimentarnos para vivir mejor" in the United States and Mexico) can be effective. Evaluations of "Salsa Sabor y Salud" and of "Sensible Solutions" have demonstrated positive results (although improvements will be needed over time). Friedman reemphasized that collaboration is the only way to obtain support and effectiveness from industry interventions.

Enrique de la Madrid, Mexican Council of Food Product Manufacturers (Consejo Mexicano de la Industria de Productos de Consumo) and member of the Alliance for a Healthy Life (Alianza por una Vida Saludable, a group of seven industry associations that have initiated a response to the obesity issue), presented his views on the food industry's role in obesity prevention. Alianza por una Vida Saludable is composed of associations linked to consumer and food products, health, restaurant, retail, and media associations. De la Madrid agreed with Friedman regarding the importance of partnering with groups like the Alliance for a Healthy Life—which works collaboratively with industry, government, and society. The Alliance adheres to the following principles: (1) an appropriate weight and energy balance are important to good health, and nutrition should be balanced, varied, wholesome, and sufficient; (2) education on nutritional habits and healthy lifestyles is essential; (3) there are no good or bad foods but healthier or not so healthy behaviors; (4) the food industry needs to contribute to improving public health by offering a broader, healthier range of food products such as those with less amounts of fats, sugars, and salt; and (5) collaboration among the stakeholders is critical to the Alliance's objectives. Hand-in-hand with these principles is the fact that physical activity should be an essential aspect of a healthy lifestyle.

De la Madrid advocates changing food and nutrition policies as another obesity prevention strategy. For example, changes in labels should reflect revisions in the product formulation so that consumers are informed of nutritional improvements or potential health benefits from consuming specific foods. In de la Madrid's opinion, the food industry should develop logos with standards for health, nutritional details, and functional information. He cautions, though, that companies should be attentive to the Mexican legal framework, cultural values, ideologies, and other societal idiosyncrasies before implementing strategies that have worked in other countries.

According to de la Madrid, the food industry supports efforts to improve the quantity and quality of physical activity, and also supports the idea of regulations and restrictions in advertisement; however, in his view industry experts must participate in the making of such regulations as part of developing an effective, multidisciplinary effort in modifying the national policy. De la Madrid also insisted that solutions be based on scientific data rather than on opinions or social pressures. In addition to developing healthier foods, the industry could also collaborate with the government to spread messages about healthy lifestyles.

Plenary discussions on the value of government regulation versus industry self-regulation revealed divergent opinions. The discussions highlighted government regulations schemes that were effective for public health (such as those for the tobacco industry or for environmental contaminants) but industry representatives, who favor self-regulation, did not welcome the idea. The majority of the participants agreed that where multifactorial aspects come into play—culture, environment, product choices, marketing practices—collective responsibility, collaboration, and partnerships are crucial. Evaluating the risk factors and trying to address each one, making progress in all fronts would be the best approach. This opinion was supported especially by industry members, who insisted that the much-needed national policy in Mexico should include industry participation.

In a nutshell, participants from industry supported the idea of collaborative efforts and self-regulation as a starting point, followed by government regulations when appropriate. As an example of collaboration in the United States, the American Beverage Association and the Alliance for a Healthier Generation recently made a special announcement that through the participation of the American Heart Association and the William Clinton Foundation, the beverage industry, including Coca Cola, Pepsi Cola, and Cadbury Schweppes, will voluntarily restrict the selection of school products; for example elementary schools will only sell water and 8-oz. portion servings of nonfat milk and certain juices. This unprecedented announcement is an excellent example of industry self-regulation and collaboration. A second example is that of a successful industry–government collaboration. Nieves Cruz, the Robert Wood Johnson Foundation, talked about the communication campaign "Salud te Recomienda" or "The Health Department Recommends," which is the first Puerto Rican public policy effort on guiding the public on how to make food choices. The resulting public awareness has created changes in restaurants, including healthier options in menus. According to Cruz, this is a real success story of collaboration that could, and should, be applied elsewhere.

Collaboration with industry was also addressed by Working Group III. Members of the Working Group III generally believed that a dialogue should be opened with industry to address media educational campaigns, policy changes, norms and regulation, and other environmental changes. They also agreed that communication with the media and the public should be carefully planned and executed in order to avoid public panic. In the United States, industry has been able to expand its portfolios and is now offering products lower in energy density and higher in micronutrients contents. Friedman emphasized that there needs to be a recognition that this change has been accomplished via many concerted efforts, dialog, and research and that the community should not expect a sudden change in the products in supermarket shelves but a gradual one that will come only through collaboration. De la Madrid noted that the progress made thus far in Mexico was demonstrated by the development of a nutrition guidance reached by consensus (see Figure 3-1), labeling proposals made to the public health authority and industry efforts to broaden the range of products.

Pate indicated that the role of the food industry can also be extrapolated to the electronic entertainment industry as they contribute to the physical activity levels of children. This is an area that unfortunately lags far behind in terms of translating research into advocacy even though there is evidence that reducing exposure to electronic entertainment has a strong impact on behavior and body composition of children. The electronic entertainment industry, he proposed, should follow some guidelines or regulations to prevent obesity.

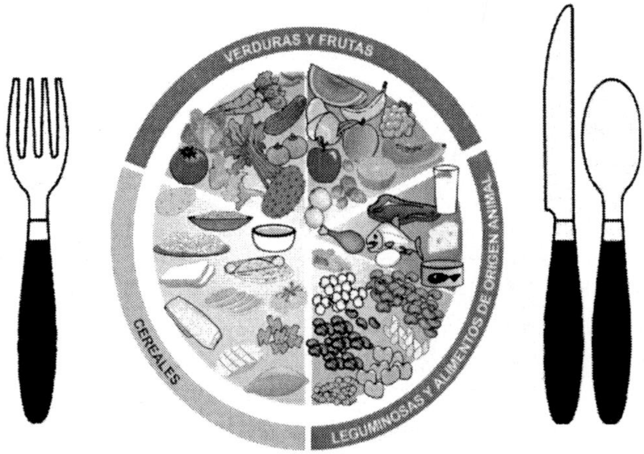

FIGURE 3-1 El plato del bien comer. Dietary guidelines.
SOURCE: Norma Oficial Mexicana (2005).

Communications industry. Robert Valdez, Univision Communications Corporation's "Salud es Vida: ¡Enterate!" health campaign, concurs that media has a significant role in disseminating health messages. In his view, there is a need to engage community leaders and youth in designing interventions, especially those that entail media messages combined with community-based activities. "Salud es Vida: ¡Enterate!," is an example of what the communications industry can do in the prevention of obesity and its consequences.

Univision Communications Corporation is composed of a radio network, three television networks, an Internet portal (the largest Spanish-language portal in the United States), and three music labels and owns and operates stations across the United States, including Puerto Rico. Univision decided to engage in a healthy lifestyle-oriented health promotion and disease prevention campaign called "Salud es Vida: ¡Enterate!" as a five-year corporate commitment to improving and protecting the health of its audience. ¡Enterate! developed partnerships with voluntary organizations (e.g., the American Heart Association, the American Diabetes Association), governmental agencies (e.g., the National Cancer Institute, Office of Minority Health), private philanthropies (e.g., the Kaiser Family Foundation), and health profession associations to develop and deliver state of the art healthcare advice and recommendations. Partner organizations assisted in developing key messages and consumer materials and operated telephone assistance lines in English and Spanish for Univision audiences across the nation. ¡Enterate! helped partner organizations build national and regional infrastructure to assist Spanish-speaking clients that had previously been unavailable. Univision reaches over 98 percent of the Spanish-speaking population of the United States. Yet, this campaign has received relatively little commercial sponsorship because the campaign does not engage in direct advertising of its sponsors. ¡Enterate! features a national calendar of health promotion and disease prevention messages with themes changing on a monthly basis. These messages are brought to life using recognizable Univision entertainment and news talent in the form of public service announcements, sponsored vignettes, a weekly radio call-in program, news segments, and a quarterly half-hour television special. In addition, each local station (there are more than 52 television stations and approximately 60 radio stations) has a public affairs officer whose job is to engage the local community in addressing a locally identified health or healthcare issue or concern. On the news side of the business and on the public service side, there is control over the design and development of the messages. However, on the entertainment programming side, there is a need to work with Mexican, Brazilian, and other Latin American television industries that supply the bulk of U.S.-viewed tele-novelas and other entertainment programming. In Valdez's opinion, by influencing the production of entertainment programming that supports healthy lifestyle and anti-violence messages the public health community can expand the reach of health promotion and disease prevention messages. Otherwise, viewers are apt to encounter unhealthful portrayals in entertainment programs. The establishment of the Mexican Alliance for a Healthy Life is an important development for a binational effort and could assist Univision work with Mexican business and media corporations to craft entertainment shows that support healthy lifestyle portrayals.

Frederick Trowbridge mentioned the Coalition for Healthy Children, a program of the Ad Council to develop consistent messages for dissemination by the U.S. media corporations. Friedman added that this is a good example of collaboration with industry and that the approach of donating some of the public service announcement times to air this campaign rather than asking for financial contributions would be much more agreeable to industry leaders.

Role of the Public Sector

Laura Khan, Centers for Disease Control and Prevention (CDC), presented a U.S. perspective on the role of the public sector by summarizing the CDC's primary role as the lead U.S. public health institution in providing surveillance and monitoring of disease, conducting research, and disseminating information. The CDC is also involved in public-policy efforts, whether for marketing and media, legislation, or partnerships.

The CDC uses an approach that encompasses all societal levels and disciplines. Historically, prevention of disease has been the foundation of all strategies from increasing physical activity, decreasing sedentary behavior, and promoting sound nutrition. Major efforts during the last five years have been in the development of environmental policy in regards to built environment which focuses on community design as well as access to places such as parks, sidewalks and public transportation. However, with the fast progression of the obesity epidemic, the CDC recognizes that prevention measures should be supplemented with control strategies. This conceptual redirection of the CDC's approach has resulted in two new goals: (1) preventing excess weight gain and (2) achieving and maintaining healthy weight loss and weight maintenance.

Recognizing that the interventions for achieving energy balance are not yet fully based on scientific evidence, the CDC is focusing on various areas of both basic and translational research. For example, the CDC is collaborating with the Robert Wood Johnson Foundation and other partners to determine indicators of obesity prevention and control for national, state, and community levels at specific intervention levels. Another area of great interest is the evaluation of interventions. The CDC recognizes that before spending vital resources in implementation of interventions, researchers should develop a systematic process to evaluate their efficacy; this is especially true when evidence data on the effectiveness of interventions are not ideal. Researchers have proposed an initial set of criteria so that potential interventions, which will be evaluated further, are selected more rigorously; the funding organizations should participate in the evaluation process. According to Khan, conducting collaborative projects between the INSP and the CDC, in particular in the area of surveillance and evaluation of programs, would be a beneficial step forward in establishing a U.S.–Mexico binational program.

Khan said that in addition to surveillance and evaluation, there are other critical areas where partnerships could be beneficial. The recent Keystone Forum on Foods Away from Home (contracted by the U.S. Food and Drug Administration) is a model of collaboration between industry, academia, and government that has resulted in a plan of action with recommendations to the industry on informing consumers and increasing availability of lower calorie foods and menu items. This plan of action was set by the industry rather than by a government authority and, according to Khan, has demonstrated the industry's commitment toward offering a healthier diet. In the international arena, a CDC–PAHO (PanAmerican Health Organization) initiative assists people with individualized dietary assessments and recommendations based on their BMI; there is also a Food Stamps Pilot Study aiming to lower the caloric content of diets in low-income populations.

Obviously, as part of this approach to obesity prevention and control one should not dismiss parents as role models. In this sense, there is a lack of specific recommendations from the public sector on communication and educational strategies that will ensure appropriate behaviors of parents as role models or educators. One option being considered at the CDC is a strategy located at work sites. This could be a golden opportunity to educate and involve employers in the family responsibility for promoting children's good health, including the benefits of physical activity as well as healthy eating choices for the family. Not only would employees and their families benefit, but employers could have a healthier workforce and possibly could save insurance costs.

Some areas where the public sector has a role in preventing obesity are controversial. For example, the value of BMI screening of youths at schools is controversial because of potential unintended, harmful consequences. The issue of surveillance at federal, state, and community levels also has become part of the debate. Although there is surveillance at the federal level, there is a gap in surveillance at state and community levels; the CDC is considering the value of pursuing such a surveillance as well as feasible options for conducting them.

Khan discussed other controversies (e.g., those surrounding the cost of preventative programs). In her view, which was supported by many others, cost-effectiveness analysis will be very useful for leaders in government (or other sectors) to make decisions about investing in programs on obesity prevention and control. As an example, Mendoza mentioned that in California the cost of obesity estimates are up to $24 billion; not surprisingly this is the driving force to act urgently. Unfortunately, Khan commented, the current investment from the U.S. Congress in CDC activities related to obesity prevention in statewide programs is less than $0.20 per person compared with the tobacco program investments of $2.75–3.50 dollars per person. Realistically, cost estimates for preventing the epidemic are $5.00–7.00 dollars per person. Programs to prevent and control obesity may be better justified by conducting cost-effectiveness analysis. It is likely that decision makers on both sides of the border will pay attention to this kind of analysis (e.g., the cost of treating diabetes or heart disease versus implementing obesity preventative measures) so that better budget strategies that are economical and beneficial for public health are developed. Such high costs calls for financial support from government but also from foundations, corporations, or the community, Khan also noted.

Mauricio Hernández, INSP, discussed the role of the public sector from a Mexican perspective. His discussion highlighted differences among European Union, United States, and Mexican systems on public mechanisms for changing public policies. For example, Hernández pointed out that in the European Union as well as in the United States, civil society is empowered to demand restrictions on potentially harmful activities. He emphasized important differences at the legislative level; in the United States and European Union the reelection of congressmen ensures that electoral interests are considered by decision makers. In contrast, in Mexico, legislators cannot be elected for a second term, which results in a system that weakens the public's influence in the policy-making process; in this manner, elements of a healthy society might be dismissed easily. These differences are critical in understanding how strategies to improve public health might need to be adapted to the political (or other) framework in each country.

According to Hernández, the perception that public health prevents business and industry development is no longer justifiable; a successful example is the economic gains achieved by industry after revisions to environmental laws. Hernández's view is that, in order for the government to maintain its commitment to promoting and sustaining public health, Mexico needs a public health system that includes development, implementation, and enforcement of regulations as well as the power of litigation (i.e., the power to sue in court to enforce a law or demand justice). To support this perspective he recommends developing laws that protect those who are unable to decide for themselves, for example, laws to protect children from making bad dietary choices. The laws also must be based on undeniable scientific evidence in support of a regulation. In addition to scientific evidence, the political will and resources to develop, implement, and enforce such laws are critical elements for effective regulation. Failure to gain political will often constitutes a limitation in the Mexican context, although lack of scientific evidence and resources also can impede progress in policy making. In the case of obesity, there is scientific evidence that the problem is real; but even so, progress towards a set of interventions is a challenge because there is no clear evidence on the association between specific factors and risk of obesity. Hernández reiterated the complexity of the risk factors associated with obesity and the multidisciplinary and multisectorial nature of the solutions needed.

According to Hernández some of the solutions for obesity prevention in children include the following:

- Regulatory interventions at the regional, state, and national level.
- Market controls through the implementation of government subsidies or other.
- Evaluation of interventions.
- Collaborative interventions with the food industry.
- Research support.
- Surveys of obesity prevalence with adequate indicators.
- Interventions at the school level.
- Food-marketing regulations.

Mexico has had great successes in the prevention of infectious diseases but the programs for health promotion with regard to chronic diseases have failed, and it is reflected in the high rates of obesity and diabetes, Hernández said. There is a disconnect between the existence of excellent clinics and surgeons to ensure high-quality treatments and the scarcity of effective preventative health programs, such as macro-environment changes that are more desirable than those purely based on high-quality treatments.

In summary, Hernandez believes that in a society like Mexico's, regulation should be used as a tool to ensure the health of the Mexican population. The regulatory process needs to be followed in a responsible manner and should be based on scientific findings and consider the unique Mexican societal characteristics.

Ultimately, participants believed that industry self-regulation and government regulation should be considered. Self-regulation—imposing limitations that can be explained by the desire of companies to be competitive, not only in the financial sense but also in the quality and healthy features of their products—is a complicated issue and was controversial among some participants. Even though there are many success stories from self-regulating measures taken by industry, the group also recognized that it might be challenging to transfer the self-regulatory approach to small companies, which often are not active participants in discussions regarding self-regulation. The unifying theme in the group was that collaboration among sectors and disciplines is crucial.

Role of the International Community

Agricultural research and international policies can shape the cost, and eventually consumption, of food commodities. For example, the high cost of fruits and vegetables is currently a subject of much debate and efforts are being made to lower their cost. The Consultative Group on International Agricultural Research, a consortium of agricultural institutions throughout the world (e.g., CYMMIT for corn and wheat in Mexico, the Rice Center in the Philippines, the Potato Center in Peru) has considered priorities in agricultural research. These institutions are shifting the emphasis in research toward achieving high productivity for fruits and vegetables. A particular concern is the impact of this shift on trading activities of poor producers in developing countries, which already need to meet the very strict quality demands of food markets. For example, it is not cost-effective for poor farmers to market cereals because of their high productivity and resulting low market prices. Martorell noted that agricultural research programs should ensure the participation and needs of poor producers. He also commented that the influence of agricultural policies and markets in the final prices of specific commodities and further consequences in patterns of food consumption cannot be overlooked. López agreed with this proposition and indicated that there is an opportunity to define a binational strategy that can impact international trade policies.

INFORMATION AND RESEARCH GAPS

Working Group II discussed areas where there are information gaps critical to making progress toward lessening the prevalence of obesity among children and youth. The goal of this section is to frame the information needs into a research agenda that can be translated into action. As pointed out by Arturo Jimenez, Universidad Autónoma de Baja California, in order for an obesity prevention program to succeed, more researchers from the different academic institutions and the leaders of these institutions should participate in the development of the program so that they can convey the findings to the communities. Research institutions need to maintain long-term relations with the community and strive to link research to actions.

Thomas Robinson, Stanford University, summarized the discussions of Working Group II on research needed to further progress in reversing childhood obesity. He noted that research and development on interventions needs to encompass all life stages. The group did not find a consensus on which life stages should receive greater priority; however, early childhood appeared to be one critical stage. Other stages that would benefit from further research are prenatal stages (e.g., investigating interventions that could help prevent gestational diabetes). Working Group II also related that research should focus on school-based and community-based interventions, which might be particularly effective in preventing childhood obesity. Regardless of the selection of intervention venues or life stages, industry was seen as a key player in the process to translate research findings to feasible interventions. Questions were also raised on how industry could engage in decision processes and interventions that are attuned with requests and expectations from the public and healthcare community. The two main themes identified by the working group as needing further research (summarized below) were (1) risk factors associated with childhood obesity, particularly those related to behavioral patterns, along with strategies for interventions and implementations, and (2) design and implementation of studies to evaluate the efficacy of interventions and programs to prevent childhood obesity.

Identifying Risk Factors, Interventions, and Implementation Strategies

The broad questions that need investigation are the following: What interventions and strategies will be effective in obesity prevention among Mexican–American and Mexican children? How should these interventions be implemented? What specific research designs and testing interventions are needed? The working group recognized the lack of knowledge on effective interventions as was also concluded in the IOM report *Preventing Childhood Obesity* (2005).

Although not discussed during the Working Group II session, Robinson noted the importance of evaluating the significance of potential outcomes of an intervention prior to actually conducting the study. That is, he insisted on the importance of weighing the strength of each hypothesis and whether the outcome might result in a feasible solution. For instance, investigating safety in the community as a risk factor for obesity by looking at the level of safety and of physical activity in children might not have any value because, regardless of the outcome, an increase in safety will always be pursued. Efforts in these types of studies should not be a priority. A better approach would be to design a specific intervention that increases safety and to analyze its effect on physical activity; such a study could provide information about the efficiency of the intervention and can be the basis of decisions about whether or not to implement it. To avoid futile results as in the example above, researchers should always question whether the result of the study ultimately is going to lead to changes. In connection to this, the concept of solution-oriented research as research designs that lead directly to policy or practice changes that also includes an evaluation component was supported by the Working Group II.

Behavioral Research

One area that was identified by the working group as critical is experimental behavioral research on motivation and eating behaviors. Some participants insisted that messages about the health consequences of maintaining a healthy weight are not effective incentive factors, and that sociocultural factors such as beauty, fun, wealth, and success are much more likely to lead to changes in behavior. Understanding these behavioral factors is key to develop interventions that will result in long-term diet and physical activity attitude changes. This research should be conducted with subgroups of Mexicans and Mexican Americans, differing by location (urban versus rural), by socioeconomics, esthetics, and geographic origin. Other factors to consider are the length of the acculturation process for immigrants in the United States and the migration patterns. Acculturation factors might contribute to the diet and physical activity patterns of immigrants; if this is the case, then the group noted that searching for incentives to moderate any negative effect of the acculturation factors and values of certain subgroups on populations on diet and physical activity levels would be an important focus of behavioral research.

Participants also noted that marketing research data would be a valuable resource to begin to answer the questions above and developing interventions. The use of market data for developing interventions was recommended in the 2005 IOM report *Preventing Childhood Obesity.* The difficulty in obtaining such data from food companies was raised. Access to data from marketing research firms and food, beverage, and restaurant companies is a challenge since they are not in the public domain. Some databases are available for a price but with many restrictions on the use of that information. IOM's Vivica Kraak reported limited success in receiving proprietary data from market researchers and companies to inform the IOM report on food marketing to children and youth during the two years that it took to complete. The IOM report recommended creating a mechanism for accessing marketing research data so that it can be used to develop social marketing and public education campaigns (IOM, 2006). Participants also observed that companies conducting market research for Mexico should also contribute to this endeavor.

For example, Khan noted that the company MPD (which also started the Nielsen TV Index) has data sets not only of food patterns in restaurants or at home but also from personal history surveys with information on physical activity. This is a phenomenal set of marketing data that are sponsored by industry but unfortunately are very expensive to obtain. The food industry, as their customers, could devise ways to make it more easily available. De la Madrid, representing the food industry, mentioned the formation of a research industry group for particular topics that could assess and share specific research findings as the best strategy to allow information exchange.

Behavioral research is critical and should be designed not only to describe but also to understand attitudes of consumers so that intervention development can include effective motivational factors. Research to help identify factors that increase behavioral adherence and maintenance is important but largely nonexistent. Following basic behavioral studies, researchers should conduct feasibility or pilot studies to design and test intervention strategies and to identify potential barriers and facilitators of behavior changes. These studies should be conducted before a randomized control trial to avoid pitfalls or failures in the more costly, randomized control study; to help refine designs so researchers know the parameters and factors to consider; and to identify and possibly manipulate mechanisms (often called mediators of interventions). Mediators may be characteristics such as language, sex, or origin; in essence, pilot studies increase the chances for success when the randomized trial is conducted. Although randomized control trials should be attempted, the working group recognized the challenges and expense of following control studies in a real-life scenario. In addition, the working group suggested that once there is more evidence that supports the association of specific risk factors to obesity, then a much broader testing of these interventions should be conducted in a less controlled, more real-life scenario.

Research on Other Risk Factors

At the present time, information on obesity-linked risk factors is scarce, so interventions are developed based on suggested associations between certain factors and obesity. The current guidelines, recommendations, and initiatives have been developed with the best available science, but there is not confirmation that they are the most appropriate ones. Therefore, there is a need to collect more data on risk factors so that eventually recommendations regarding interventions are stated with sufficient evidence. For example, research on the effects of dietary content, eating patterns, physical activity and inactivity levels, and patterns leading to obesity prevention and weight control in already obese children should continue to be investigated so that a clearer picture of the factors and relationships among them emerges. What is the amount of physical activity that is really needed for weight control or prevention? Are the dietary guidelines in the United States and Mexico appropriate for weight gain control or prevention? These questions remain unanswered but could be addressed through experimental studies or prospective studies with appropriate measurements.

Evaluating Interventions and Programs

An important aspect of reversing the obesity epidemic via interventions is to evaluate programs already implemented, whether in other countries or locally, with the objective of gaining knowledge from those experiences and applying that knowledge to develop improved or new strategies. For example, the design and selection of pilot studies should draw from the findings derived from other research and experiences on obesity or other health-related intervention and program implementations. Much of the discussion focused on the importance of studies for evaluation of macrolevel interventions (e.g., evaluation of governmental policies and actions such as food and nutrition regulations, taxations, trade policies, urban planning policies, dietary and physical activity guidelines, or other public health initiatives) with special emphasis on the intense activity in European countries, where they tend to favor governmental interventions more often than in North America. Evaluating their programs for efficacy and feasibility might be very beneficial for leaders in all sectors in both the United States and Mexico.

Evaluation also applies to industry's initiatives to prevent obesity. For example, evaluating the responses of consumers to voluntary industry changes (e.g., new products and packaging) will provide a deeper insight on consumer behavior. As mentioned previously, this might improve refinement of future interventions.

Ideally, when evaluating the outcomes associated with macrolevel interventions, experimental designs will be similar to the ones conducted on intervention effects except they will be conducted before and after an innovation or policy was introduced. Furthermore, cross-sectional comparisons among countries, states, communities, and schools will add value to the evaluation.

During the plenary discussions Simon Barquera, INSP, mentioned that contrary to what happens in other Latin American countries, broad educational programs in Mexico cannot be evaluated because they do not have specific goals. For example, a program for physical activity and nutrition in Chile has consistent goals in terms of obesity prevalence for the years 2010, 2015, and 2020. This is not contemplated in the Mexican programs. In addition, some of these programs have been implemented only for a very short time. Barquera concluded that the lack of consistent goals in conjunction with a short implementation period precludes program evaluation; in addition he recommended that food industry programs should also include evaluation. These findings could be shared with others in the community and serve as basis for continued program improvement.

Evaluating food programs was one of the research needs specifically discussed by Mexican participants. Hernandez noted that an analysis of the foods distributed by government nutrition programs such as LICONSA and DICOSA in Mexico would help researchers understand the effects of those type of foods and programs on obesity. For example, LICONSA sells subsidized foods—such as pasta and sweetened beverages—that could contribute to an increase in obesity prevalence, especially in poor and rural areas. Teresa González de Cossio, INSP, added that these programs do not distribute perishables because of long distribution distances (e.g., the main hub in Mexico City often is far from the food's destination). Better strategies for food distributions are needed. Furthermore, she said that in Mexico weight for age is used to evaluate malnutrition and eligibility for participation in food programs; the use of this indicator might erroneously include in these programs children who do not suffer from malnutrition. Various evaluations of nutrition programs in the United States suggest that their effects on the propensity of obesity are either beneficial or neutral; however, analysts note that many of the studies were not designed to assess the programs for their effects on obesity and therefore better study designs for evaluating these programs are needed.

OPPORTUNITIES FOR COLLABORATION: A BINATIONAL, COMMON AGENDA

This section addresses the ultimate objective of this workshop—to explore opportunities for collaboration between the United States and Mexico with the common objective of preventing progress of the obesity epidemic among Mexican and Mexican–American children and youth on both sides of the border. Sepúlveda reminded the audience that, in addition to positive examples of collaborative research, the IOM's *Preventing Childhood Obesity* report provides an extraordinary example and incentive to adapt those recommendations in Mexico and to follow closely the changes in obesity among the Mexican population in the United States after interventions recommended might be implemented.

This section is organized as follows. Working Group III's central proposal regarding a binational program is followed by some specific areas in which collaboration would be mutually beneficial. The summary of the presentation by Eileen Kennedy, Tufts University, highlights examples of collaboration among different sectors and levels.

Proposed Collaborations

Working Group III proposed the creation of a joint U.S.–Mexico Obesity Prevention Task Force as a cost-effective, multisectorial initiative. Some participants proposed that the task force could be expanded to include Canada, creating a North American Task Force. The responsibilities of the task force as summarized by Working Group III are listed in Box 3-1.

BOX 3-1 U.S.–Mexico Joint Obesity Prevention Task Force: Responsibilities

According to Working Group III, the responsibilities of an obesity prevention task force would include

- Develop a strategy to prevent obesity.
- Promote an obesity agenda, including a specific timeline and responsibilities.
- Promote policies and norms that will allow environmental modifications, such as schools, worksites, cities, and others.
- Develop an educational strategy in accordance with the previously stated policies and general agenda.

Specific activities identified by Working Group III as potential collaborative elements of a binational agenda in preventing childhood obesity are advocacy, funding, labor force training, scientific research, program evaluation, and ensuring consistency in programs and messages. Specific examples of collaborative elements suggested by individual participants are explained further in Box 3-2. Communications among task force members could be facilitated through conferences and the Internet so that the information on obesity prevention can be included in ongoing scientific and programmatic exchanges.

Collaborations that Work: Activities at Tufts University Friedman School of Nutrition Science and Policy

As mentioned above, Kennedy highlighted examples of collaboration among different sectors (e.g., industry, government, schools) with a common goal of a healthier environment and examined three different levels that have experienced collaborative success—community, national, and international.

Community Level

The development of collaborative strategies at the community level are based on three assumptions: the prevention of overweight and obesity is complex, small but sustainable changes occur over time, and healthy diet and physical activity are necessary components of obesity prevention. The community-level work is based on multidimensional strategies that combine the public and private sectors; however, perhaps work on the community level also needs newer paradigms to embrace because individual responsibility alone does not explain the current obesity epidemic. Although this idea is predominant among experts in this field, it is not widely shared among policy makers, who continue to put greater emphasis on individual responsibility.

An obesity intervention—called "Shape up Somerville"—was led by Tufts University in the community of Somerville, Massachusetts, and was geared toward children in first, second, and third grades; this intervention was successful in spurring environmental changes. Somerville has a low-income population and a very ethnically and racially diverse large Hispanic population composed of Mexican Americans (both recent and long-time immigrants), Guatemalans, Salvadorians, and Puerto Ricans as well as a large Asian population. Kennedy explained that the driving force behind this intervention was the realization that individual behavior change was not sufficient as a prevention strategy and that a larger environmental strategy using the social economic model was needed.

BOX 3-2 U.S.–Mexico Joint Obesity Prevention Task Force: Suggested Elements

Participants in Working Group III listed several elements for a U.S.–Mexico Joint Obesity Prevention Task Force. These were further expanded with specific examples of collaboration by individual participants and include:

Advocacy. There is an urgent need to convey the following message to the general public and more specifically to funding institutions and government—obesity is a major problem in Mexico and the United States and has major economic and health consequences. Academia, industry, and the health sector need to transmit this message with efficacy and determination using scientific data as basis. The joint U.S.–Mexico Obesity Prevention Task Force could undertake such an educational campaign.

Funding. There are funding opportunities on both sides of the border. Collaboration in identifying potentially beneficial resources will be an important endeavor. Some potential funders, alone or in partnership, might be the International Life Sciences Institute, the Pan American Heath Organization, National Institutes of Health, Conacyt, and industry.

Training of labor force. Creating of solutions requires new skills for a new and complex problem that can be addressed only through interventions at all levels and through all sectors. The Mexican labor force needs to be trained to respond to the problems of malnutrition and obesity in implementation, evaluation, and management of programs. The Mexican–American community also needs to train its healthcare providers so that they are knowledgeable about the Mexican culture and able to give guidance on lifestyles conducive to overall health and weight management.

Research. This area needs multidisciplinary, expert teamwork. Examples of research areas that could be conducted jointly are:

- Develop a system of standard instruments including growth curves, indicators of obesity that will enable comparative analysis of levels, tendencies, and health nutritional problems. Also, a joint system of indicators for other health nutritional problems that will enable comparative analysis was suggested.
- Conduct comparable surveys in the United States as well as in Mexico so data can be shared and compared.
- Extend the system to other countries in North and Central America. What is the best parameter to use that indicates childhood obesity? Is it BMI, waist circumference, abdominal obesity, or others? Or a combination of them?
- Conduct epidemiological studies in Central and North America.

continued

BOX 3-2 Continued

- Conduct studies to explore the influence of acculturation on the prevalence of childhood obesity, that is, the influence of changes in behavior that Mexican Americans experience as they integrate in the U.S. society and they adopt U.S. social norms and habits.
- Research on social norms of other countries in Europe and Australia that do not promote an obesigenic environment to evaluate their application to the United States and Mexico.
- Evaluate the cost for consumers of new products.
- Analyze cost of interventions (e.g., nutrition interventions) and cost of obesity, also taking into consideration the associated comorbidities.

Program evaluation. This area also needs multidisciplinary, expert teamwork. Examples of evaluation that could be conducted jointly are:

- Introduce measurements of obesity indicators or other health outcomes as elements of intervention and programs so they can be evaluated.
- Identify obesity prevention goals at short-, middle-, and long-term. For example, physical activity programs have been implemented in Mexico but only if they have goals can they be evaluated.
- Evaluate the effect on obesity prevalence and other health outcomes of subsidized food programs such as the Mexican Oportunidades and PrevenIMSS, and school breakfast programs or the U.S. Special Supplemental Nutrition Program for Women, Infants, and Children (WIC). As such, they should include measurements to prevent obesity.
- Evaluate the impact of the regulations and programs on obesity and other health outcomes.
- Evaluate macro-level interventions in different countries and form collaborations to share findings.

Consistency in programs and messages. As the United States and Mexico increase their cultural and commercial exchanges, actions in both countries need to occur simultaneously so that inconsistent and counterproductive policies, guidances, educational programs, and other efforts are avoided. The need for consistency applies to the many ongoing programs mentioned in the section "Specific Interventions to Prevent Obesity in Children and Youth of Mexican Origin." Examples are:

- Development of consistent propriety logos in food items so that the public associates them with a specific health benefit (e.g., a reduction of trans fatty acids content in foods).
- Harmonizations of some regulations, such as the labeling regulations.
- Health promotion messages and educational materials that reach Mexican and Mexican–American youth via radio, television, the Internet, and printed media could be adapted and shared.

Community members, healthcare providers, media, restaurants, and other private-sector groups were involved in a three-year effort to influence the children's overall activities in their homes, before school, during school, and in after-school programs. Six city departments, 86 organizations and businesses, 320 community members, and 20 restaurants were involved. The initiative included activities such as assessing breakfast foods; incorporating walk-to-school programs that were overseen by adults in the community; engaging parents; and making other changes in physical activity, food services, and curriculum in the classroom or after school. As a result, there were major modifications in school food service (e.g., additions of a la carte items and more fresh foods), curriculum recess, and after-school and at-home activities. Data from the evaluation of this program are currently being analyzed. At base line, 40 percent of the first, second, and third graders were either at-risk for or overweight. Although the evaluation analysis is still in progress, initial findings for the first three years of the intervention show a significant decrease in obesity when compared with other school rates that are increasing. This initial result of a decrease in obesity prevalence surpasses the outcome expectation, Kennedy said, which was a slow down in the increase of obesity, rather than an actual decrease. Such positive achievement shows the potential for future successes in decreasing rates of obesity with the implementation of community participatory approaches. She also noted that in order to realize all the benefits, researchers need to look beyond changes in the prevalence of obesity and factor in additional benefits, such as those from healthcare savings derived from improvements in associated diseases (e.g., asthma).

During the discussion period, many questions arose on the cost and benefits of such an intervention and on the potential increase of costs to the school and families. Kennedy acknowledged the potential for higher costs of introducing a diet higher in fruits and vegetables. She said that one interesting note was that because of the higher costs of food items, negotiations between the city government and vendors took place that finally resulted in vendors compromising profits in turn for an increase in client numbers. During plenary discussions it became clear that there is a real gap on data on cost-effectiveness of nutritional interventions.

Finally, she concluded that programs like this have an enormous potential for exploring commonalities as well as differences in U.S. and Mexican community approaches. Analyzing the data sets could provide universal lessons on unique environment situations.

National Level

National approaches that reach a much larger population are clearly desirable. One approach by Tufts University has been to implement interventions to change dietary behaviors at point of purchase. The U.S. Department of Agriculture and Tufts University in conjunction with Safeway (a nationwide supermarket chain that reaches 30 million consumers per year) have entered into a cooperative agreement to implement specific interventions. This approach—which suggests an increase in trust between the government and private sector—is based on the supermarket's historical data for motivational factors behind shopping (e.g., price, convenience, time, health). The resulting multiprong intervention includes in-store promotions, mailings, and kiosks. During the discussion period it was mentioned that an intervention like this could also be adapted in Mexico.

International Level

The International Union of Nutritional Sciences (IUNS) is a worldwide nutrition body that represents 156 different countries and various different scientific bodies. IUNS has asked Tufts University to organize a task force to identify newer paradigms for inducing public- and private-sector collaborations and to test them on countries that are more receptive to collaboration; this task force could make an enormous contribution as a model initiative for an international and bilateral collaboration.

REFERENCES

IOM (Institute of Medicine). 2005. *Preventing Childhood Obesity: Health in the Balance.* Washington, DC: The National Academies Press.

IOM. 2006. *Food Marketing to Children and Youth: Threat or Opportunity?* Washington, DC: The National Academies Press.

Norma Oficial Mexicana. 2005. NOM-043-SSA2-2005, Servicios básicos de salud. Promoción y educación para la salud en materia alimentaria. Criterios para brindar orientación.

WHO (World Health Organization). 2004. *Global Strategy on Diet, Physical Activity, and Health.* Report No. WHA57.17. [Online]. Available: http://www.who.int/gb/ebwha/pdf_files/WHA57/A57_R17-en.pdf [accessed May 7, 2006].

4

Summary and Final Remarks

SUMMARY

This section summarizes final thoughts by Reynaldo Martorell and Jeffrey Koplan; the remarks are followed by a summary of the workshop as presented by Juan Rivera.

Martorell reminded the audience of the global nature of this epidemic and that developing intervention programs entail serious consideration to the unique context within each country. For example, in Mexico, the political situation will largely determine when and how a national plan for obesity prevention in children can be initiated. It is important that national surveys on obesity continue so they can serve to increase the awareness of the epidemic. The hope is that the new government will use the data as a basis in formulating its programs. In addition to a national plan in Mexico, Martorell supports a U.S.–Mexico binational collaboration in different areas involving government, academic institutions, industries, and nongovernmental organizations (NGOs). Collaborative exchanges on research indicators, monitoring, and program efficacy and evaluation will be useful. Mechanisms for collaborative training of human resources can ensure the continuity of initiatives. The joint search for funding resources will also be beneficial; Martorell also suggested forming a small group to design an action plan for identifying potential mechanisms and funding resources.

Koplan gave some comments on the workshop discussions, focusing on the role of industry and government. Koplan emphasized the importance of alliances between industry and other partners in both the United States and

Mexico and noted that these alliances need to be carefully crafted so that they are not perceived as being driven by industry's interests and thus risk losing credibility. To develop and maintain public trust in the alliances' initiatives he recommends that industry takes a participant's role rather than a leadership role.

He reiterated the role of industry and noted that self-regulation continues to be a point of debate, but he commended the food industry on the many initiatives it already has undertaken. However, he indicated that additional questions need to be answered, such as those related to the definition of a healthy product by developing a standard label for healthier products or other mechanism. He suggested that industry has an even broader role as an advocate for all healthy lifestyle activities, for example, it could serve as an advocate for the Verb Campaign (see Appendix C for a description), whose U.S. government funding unfortunately was stopped because of priorities other than obesity prevention. One of Koplan's concerns is that the U.S. government does not invest sufficiently in prevention in general and in obesity control in particular, and such investment is required to make real progress in obesity prevention.

Koplan concluded that the role of the media should include a coherent, coordinated commitment throughout all programming to deliver a message about exercise and diet that will have much more impact than a discrete health message. Different circumstances will require carefully crafted messages depending on the communication means; for example, the nature of a message from a public health authority should be different from a more creative health message embedded in a TV show.

Workshop discussions, noted Koplan, conveyed how the profound differences in systems and cultures between Mexico and the United States could serve as lessons and result in synergistic, greater collaborative opportunities among different sectors and countries.

Juan Rivera summarized workshop discussions in more detail. Rivera reiterated the goals of the workshop and presented obesity trends in the United States (see Figure 2-1), providing a clear picture of the increase in prevalence since the 1970s. The 2005 IOM report, *Preventing Childhood Obesity: Health in the Balance,* concluded that childhood obesity is an important public health problem, both in the United States and in Mexico and that Mexican–American children are among the most affected. The complexity of the problem might be augmented in the case of Mexican–American children because of the exchange of people across the borders and the potential consequences related to shifts in culture, language, food, media, economy, and trade. The 2005 IOM report provided an enlightening review of the implications for children and society and a set of recommendations for all sectors of society to be engaged and participate in the solutions. Such a review was critical as a basis for this workshop and served to understand the nature of the problem, including risk factors. The key conclusions of the IOM report were that obesity in children is a nationwide health problem requiring a population-based prevention approach; the goal is energy balance (i.e., healthful eating behaviors and regular physical activity); society changes at all levels are needed; and multiple sectors and stakeholders should participate for programs to be successful. According to the report, a set of associated and interrelated factors play an important role in determining the energy balance and they relate to all sectors and disciplines (i.e., individuals, communities, and macrolevels); interventions at all of these levels will be the key to reversing the epidemic (see Figure 2-7, the ecological model of obesity).

In addition to the IOM report, an international framework for childhood obesity prevention was developed by the World Health Organization–Food and Agriculture Organization (WHO–FAO) through a group of experts as part of a broad task addressing diet, nutrition, and chronic disease prevention. The evidence on factors responsible for obesity were carefully evaluated and were the basis for the global strategy on diet, physical activity, and health approved by the World Health Assembly in 2004 (Mexico was a participant). Two other documents about obesity in Mexican and Mexican–American children and youth (see Appendixes B and C) were used as basis for the discussions in this meeting.

It is clear that obesity is a serious health problem in Mexico (see Figures 2-5 and 2-6). As in the United States, the obesity prevalence is growing for children under 5 years old (based on the trends in data from 1988 and 1999), and it is expected to grow even more. In addition, data from INSP show that children engage in physical activity for only one to two hours a day, but the time they spend watching television or playing videos is double that amount. Although the authors of the papers in the Appendix B found no published information from surveys regarding barriers against physical activity engagement among Mexican children, U.S. data suggest that barriers such as expense, transport, availability, and personal safety are more substantial in the Hispanic population than for whites or African Americans.

Dietary habits in Mexico have changed, where the consumption of meat, fruits, vegetables, and milk is giving way to an increased intake of refined carbohydrates, soda, and fats. For instance, as much as 56 percent of Mexican children consume fewer than 100 grams of fruit and vegetables per day, and only 8 percent consume the recommended amount of 400 grams per day. Interventions related to diet should focus on those factors that shape food and beverage consumption at different levels—policy making, marketing, product placement and price, cultural values, economic factors, public policies, production, distribution and promotion of food, individual and developmental factors, as well as those factors related to family and home, school and peers, neighborhood, and community. The key stakeholders involved in any intervention are families, schools, communities, healthcare, industry, media, and government.

The roles of the various sectors were discussed by experts representing public and private sectors in Mexico and the United States. Participants discussed that among the public sector, the healthcare sector should assume responsibility for assuring a healthy environment by leading in the development of a national prevention plan and coordinating interventions with other relevant sectors. In addition, all stakeholders should participate in developing evidence-based regulations. Congress should enact legislation that creates a healthy environment and the appropriate government bodies should allocate funds for obesity prevention research.

Areas identified in discussions where the participation of the private sector would be of benefit are (1) forming public–private partnerships; (2) offering a broader range of healthier foods (those with less sodium, few calories, and reduced quantities of fat and trans fatty acids); (3) providing consumer information; (4) implementing marketing strategies that encourage children to make healthy choices; (5) engaging in advocacy and dialogue; and (6) funding research and sharing information, for example, market surveys data.

With regard to the role of the community, developing obesity prevention initiatives, especially those that involve youth participation, would be a critical component of an obesity prevention agenda. The school environment was recognized as needing significant improvements, and the community could play a role in this respect.

Rivera also summarized the discussions of the three working groups. Working group I examined common themes and factors by comparing the differences and similarities of obesity prevention between the United States and Mexico. The two countries differ in that Mexico, unlike the United States, is undergoing a drastic change in dietary habits as well as facing the double burden of under- and over-nutrition. However, as far as similarities, the group identified the following:

- Childhood obesity is a major public health problem.
- There is an urgent need for action at all levels.
- The evidence on childhood obesity determinants is scarce.

Working Group II discussed data gaps and concluded that research is needed at all life stages. The following were general themes for a research agenda proposed by Working Group II:

- Continued research on risk factors especially those related to behavior but also on the dietary habits, nutrient composition of food, and physical activity patterns that lead to obesity prevention and weight control. Potential mediator factors should also be investigated. Effective interventions that place special emphasis on motivation for health-related behaviors could also be pursued.

- Research on evaluation of interventions on a macro level (e.g., evaluation of governmental policies and initiatives as well as of private-sector initiatives).

Working Group III explored actions implemented, opportunities, challenges, and barriers. The group concluded that although interventions are being implemented in many fronts, evaluations of the efficacy of the interventions are lacking. Unfortunately, there is also no sense of urgency and the public in general is unfamiliar with the economical and health consequences that obesity incurs. In addition, to reverse the perception that the task is too complex, multilevel and multifactorial interventions should be conducted in an environment of trust among the different sectors, including the public. A clear, detailed research agenda is also needed to promote evidence-based interventions.

The working group explored the opportunities for binational collaborative research and identified the importance of identifying binational funding mechanisms. A clear proposal evolved for the creation of an Obesity Prevention Task Force for Mexico in which the government has the leadership but also involves representatives of relevant stakeholders such as government, industry, civil society, and academia. An immediate goal of the task force would be to develop a national childhood obesity prevention plan that would include policies, norms, and regulations for preventing obesity; strategies for changing environmental conditions that promote obesity; communication plans for promoting behavioral change; and a plan for coordinating all of the proposed strategies. Mexico could draw from the U.S. experience and from the findings in the 2005 IOM report, *Preventing Childhood Obesity: Health in the Balance.* Additionally, results from the ENSANUT 2006 survey will demonstrate trends in obesity and could be used to increase awareness of the epidemic and to help foster a sense of urgency for action.

Binational collaborations could include sharing media-based health promotion content from radio, television, Internet, and printed media to reach Mexican and Mexican–American children; establishing guidelines for appropriate marketing targeted at children and youth; and sharing educational materials adapted for Mexican culture.

Furthermore, binational collaborations would be invaluable to (1) strengthen ongoing scientific research and programmatic exchanges; (2) compare survey findings; (3) exchange results from intervention evaluations; (4) share lessons from programs, strategies, and actions; (5) assist in training human resources with new, appropriate skills, needed to address the epidemic; and (6) explore funding strategy mechanisms.

Final Remarks

Jaime Sepúlveda

Mr. Secretary, please allow me to bridge protocol and start speaking in English so we can communicate better to our visitors from the States. I think a short introduction of Dr. Frenk will serve to help understand why it is that we feel a special privilege in Mexico in having people who come from academia move into the public sector as major decision makers; he is open and welcoming of this kind of workshop that provides the evidence. Dr. Frenk is an M.D. who also holds a Ph.D. from Michigan on healthcare organizations and sociology and in 1987 was the founding director of the National Institute of Public Health. We feel indeed that he is a member of the academic community. He is also a member of the IOM—as a foreign associate, we are not called members, we are foreign associates, it sounds distinguishing, actually. There is also a long-standing collaboration between IOM and Mexican institutions. Something like 13 years ago, Julio Frenk and Harvey Fineberg promoted an IOM–Mexican Academy of Medicine workshop on the impact of NAFTA (North American Free Trade Agreement) on our Health Services; we also had Canadian colleagues in that workshop, after which a report came out. That is just to tell you that there is a long-standing experience of collaboration with IOM and American universities on issues that are of common interest; and certainly childhood obesity is one of the largest health problems that we share.

The attitude from the main authorities of the health sector in Mexico toward evidence-based health policy is well established and, quite frankly, we feel proud about having had that not only with Julio but also with his predecessors; it is almost a quarter of a century of a tradition of having M.D.'s with Ph.D.'s very much into research and linking research results into health policy. It is going to be hard to shift.

The issue is that in the results of the National Nutrition Surveys, the first one in 1988, malnutrition was seen as the largest public health problem, but the obesity problem was increasing. Ten, eleven years later, with the second National Nutrition Survey, the obesity problem was discovered in all its magnitude, a problem that grew impressively, more than in the United States at any moment, and which turned on all the alarms. In 1999 and in 2000, when the results were made public, we remained with the alarms on, but nothing else happened. I think that the first necessary step was to have the information, but this is not enough, we have to move on to public policies. In Mexico we have the big paradox of having women of reproductive age who are obese and anemic, and we have also another cruel paradox, that of obese parents and malnourished children. That is, I believe, unacceptable.

In Mexico we have managed to decrease a great deal of malnutrition in children with national programs against poverty. We have started to work on the deficiency of micronutrients when the other problem shows up, and we still have not done anything. If we will do an evaluation of it on the economic impact, along with the other riders of the apocalypses that accompany it—hypertension, cardiovascular disease, and diabetes—then I think that we will realize that these four riders are imposing big amounts of money in the public and private healthcare sectors and lots of suffering in human beings, of course. A better estimation of the economic costs of this salient epidemic still remains to be incorporated in the agenda so that we can realize the urgency of public and private investment to face this emergency. I believe that a conclusion derived from the studies from IOM, WHO, CDC, and others, is that one will never have all the evidence one would like to act upon, nevertheless, there is already enough evidence and successful experiences at local, state, and national levels of action that could have an impact. We have to acknowledge that, unlike vaccination programs or some other programs treating infectious diseases, the reward for the effort will take time. What we do now, will be seen, if we are lucky, in one or two decades, and for this reason it might not be attractive for politicians to take difficult measures, having confrontation, for something they will not see results in during their political lives; nevertheless, it is an absolute responsibility as government employees to start taking actions in this regard. Mr. Secretary, we have a good investment in information. Soon we will have the results from the National Health Survey; the nutrition part of the last seven states will soon be picked up, and in two months we will have preliminary results. I believe we can incorporate that information in order to take public political measures. I think that Juan Rivera, in his magnificent report, stated very clearly that there are several specific steps to take in the next few months that will lead us to leave a legacy from this administration, along with other legacies that it will leave, for those who will follow us. With this short summary and thanking again all our friends from IOM, Linda Meyers, Vivica Kraak, and Maria Oria and to those who participated in those brilliant reports from the IOM, many thanks. With their work they are saving us a huge amount of work; you have distilled scientific evidence for us, and we do not have to reinvent the wheel. Many of the policies, along with the evidence supporting them, will serve us to adapt and adopt some of the policies recommended there for the different sectors involved in this complex issue. Dr. Frenk, I would like to give you the floor.

Julio Frenk

I noticed that when Jaime spoke in Spanish more people put on headphones, the worrisome thing was that several of the Mexicans put on headphones, too. At that point I decided to vividly break with protocol and speak in English, very briefly because I know you are at the end of a long work session, and this is a beautiful city that you probably would enjoy visiting, this is the City of Eternal Spring. It is really a great pleasure, first of all to meet again many good friends who have come to this seminar, and as Jaime said, I am a member, at least we are called foreign and not alien, associates we should not go [inaudible] but I am one of the three foreign associates of the IOM in Mexico, Jaime is another one, so this is both an opportunity to participate in the activities of the Institute, to continue what has been an enriching series of exchanges that I keep with the Institute, and I want to thank Mauricio Hernández again for providing the venue where I can learn. Hopefully that helps me to do my job in a better manner. We continually have seminars at the Institute where the policy makers at the Ministry of Health come, and we meet for an afternoon like now and discuss lots of input on priority issues. Certainly the one you have chosen for this seminar is a top priority. It is a silent epidemic, probably one of the clearest examples of the double burden of disease and risk factors. The fact that we still have not completely overcome the traditional old scourges of malnutrition and yet, even though we have made a lot of progress but there are still pockets, among poor people, among indigenous populations. Without having completely overcome the old problems, we now face the problems of the wealthier societies in the world, and this is the nature of the epidemiological transition in countries like Mexico, that we are always faced with that double agenda. The meeting is very timely because we are very soon going to have the results of this major survey that will provide us a third point in time. If, as Juan was already anticipating, the results show a further deterioration of the situation in terms of obesity and overweight it is a great opportunity to raise public awareness and indeed in the face of the change of administration in seven months it could well be placed as a top priority for policy making in the health arena in the future.

This is the toughest of the issues, when one looks at sins representing emergent risks to health, the one dealing with food intake and the balance with exercise is by far the toughest. Tobacco is a black-and-white situation, even one puff is harmful. You do not have to discuss a lot, it is clearly a risk to health, and you can have very clear cut interventions: rising taxes, forbidding publicity, etc.; the policy package is clear cut because the risk is clear cut. Alcohol begins to get a little bit more complex because there are certain levels of consumption that are harmless and at some levels there is even benefit; still, alcohol is not vital for sustaining life. But when you come to issues of nutrition then you are really into an area where the complex questions, by far, come because food is not only not harmful, not only beneficial, it is essential for sustaining life, so the issues become much more difficult, and I like the title of Jeff Koplan's report, the balance, I mean. The question here is the search for balance but it makes the policy debate much more difficult; the same policy packages do not apply to each of these three areas of emerging risks: tobacco, alcohol consumption, and excessive or imbalance food intake. As I said, by far this is the most difficult one. This is probably a case where we absolutely need to have evidence-based policy; we run into the temptation of pointing fingers, of trying to identify villains, and breaking lines of communication and go for more ideological decisions rather than scientifically derived evidence, but we can really cause a lot of harm.

For me, this exercise that you have done for the last two days is a clear example of how do we better build that evidence base. Let me tell you, not the only example, there are many examples but this shows the value of making long-term capacity investments. This thing here did not exist 20 years ago, and it is taking 20 years to build not only the physical infrastructure but specially the human infrastructure to reach this capacity we now have, for example, to generate this high-quality survey; the Institute is constantly involved in providing evidence based in evaluating public policies and in Mexico, I think, this is a clear example of the need to do long-term investment on intellectual capital building in developing countries. It is countries like Mexico that need evidence based, even more than the richer countries. The fact that we can even at all have this discussion is a testimony of the wisdom of particularly Dr. Guillermo Soberon, who happens to be the third foreign associate of IOM in Mexico; when he was minister, 20 years ago, he decided to start this Institute of Public Health, and now we are ripening the fruits that were sowed some many, many years ago. I am very glad to see Enrique de la Madrid because his father was the president at that point and came here to dedicate the buildings and the laboratories for the Center for Infectious Diseases. At that point, Mexico was in a very serious economic shape, oil prices, contrary to what is happening now, have dropped, we were in the mist of a major financial crisis, and yet there was a government that has the vision to say, "You know, it is exactly when you are facing constraints of that sort that you need to invest in research." I am very happy to see one more fruit of those seeds that were sowed then; we need that evidence to orient the policies that we have.

In the topic of obesity, we have two main policy instruments: the first is health protection, the other is health promotion. Health protection we interpreted as the set of tools to protect people from passive exposure to different risks, particularly regulatory mechanisms and health promotion to enhance or diminish exposure when that exposure is active. We need to use those tools in a thoughtful manner; the first one is the stick and the other is the carrot. The first one is all the regulatory framework; we have done enormous efforts in this administration to modernize our agency that does a lot of the regulation. We used to have an area in the center bureaucracy of the Secretary responsible for generating risks regarding air pollution, water pollution, food contamination of various sorts, so we regulatory role for almost everything because almost everything can be a risk to health. Now we have an independent, autonomous agency, a little bit like the Food and Drug Administration, except it also has elements of the Environmental Protection Agency and Occupational Safety and Health Administration. We set standards for occupation and environmental exposures, although we do not enforce them but we do set the standards. It is a very important agency called Federal Commission for Protection against Health Risks, that is actually its name so we are emphasizing the concept of protection and the idea is protecting people from risks factors where exposure is passive. Just by breathing, one brings risks to health, or a very major passive exposure which is information for example to publicity, so through the action of that, for example, we have completely ban now publicity on tobacco; for issues of labeling and marketing, we can actually use that policy too. We have found great merit in frameworks for self-regulation. As you know Mexico has made a major transition towards full-fledged democracy, and we believe in collaborating with all social sectors. In fact, with many of the major industrial groups, including Con-Mexico, with Enrique de la Madrid, and the individual companies that form it, we are trying to create a framework that is based on collaboration. The value of self-regulation is that it is not a soft government because self-regulation is based on trust and those that engage in self-regulation know that if the trust if bridged, then the response from the government has to be even tougher than pure regulation. That has been our philosophy and it has worked on a number of arenas.

The other policy instrument that we have is health promotion, to enhance people's capacity to reduce their exposures, empower people to reduce their exposures where the exposure is active, as a function of choices that are made and behaviors that are engaged. Here, of course, our great tool is health promotion, just a couple of things that have happened, a whole new Official Mexican Norm (Norma Oficial Mexicana), in Mexico we have a standard-setting approach for a number of areas that have to be participatory. It took us almost four years of dialog, with all the actors, the research community, the NGOs, the activists, industry, and we finally came up with a new standard for nutritional orientation, and I would like to encourage the National Institute and maybe in this collaboration to actually begin thinking on an evaluative research on what happens; we did four years of huge process investment because these things get published, then all social groups can send comments, any kind of comment; once it has been commented on, all those comments are processed, every single comment has to be responded. In this case, this was probably, from the many standards that we issue, the one that generated the largest amount of interaction with society. I think we finally have come up with the didactic tool, which is the nutritional dish, no longer the pyramid but the dish, which emphasizes the idea of balance and so forth; but we should monitor what happens because once you put that out if behavior does not change, it ends up being just one more document; this will not be good.

The other big initiative has been a program with the Ministry of Education, which we call Healthy Education, and that by the way has the participation of two private philanthropies: Banamex and Fundación Arronte. We have formed a special fund to promote health-promoting activities in schools, including now tobacco- and smoke-free schools, and part of the issues, there is nutritional attention, improving the nutritional quality of the food sold in the schools. Those are a few of the things, but I think we have a long way to go, particularly on the health promotion, which is actually the toughest part because it involves changing perceptions, changing behaviors, and part of the problem of the perception, is the risk perception, the fact that people tend to have very distorted assessments of relative risks.

A new instrument that we will develop is a new initiative that is called Take Measures, in the double sense of measuring your waist and then taking some measures in your life; we are distributing this paper strip to measure your waist and then it has different colors. If you are in the red you really ought to begin thinking about what you eat and how much exercise you do. But this is, I think, a long road ahead and particularly, shifting the perception of the population is going to be our biggest challenge. This is why, concluding, I really welcome the international collaboration, this is a field where obviously the epidemic of obesity is very much linked to forces of globalization, in fact some people have spoken of this new concept of globesity, meaning linking obesity to globalization, globesity, so the answer of global problems has to be global solutions and the best tool we have in global solutions is cooperation, dialog. I firmly believe we need to create knowledge-based international public good research, and I am very happy to see that there is a research agenda, but then also what Jaime said, the constant point is that, well you have just enough evidence, and you have to continue building the research evidence doing a lot of evaluative research to see if what you are doing is actually working. We need processes to share learning lessons. We were just talking with Jeff, can Mexico take the leap? Are we condemned to follow the same path of the non-Hispanic Whites or other populations in the United States? Can we learn something for Mexican-origin populations in the United States and here? Is there a way of, by engaging in a process of learning what regulatory measures or health promotion measures would avoid us the pain? We have done that on tobacco. We do not have to go through the same set of steps before we act, but as I said before, this is a much more complex area, it has much more cultural underpinnings, societal underpinnings, but I believe we should do learn from each other to adapt and adopt what has proven to work in other countries, what is obviously culturally, financially, feasible in our country.

The other reason for welcoming this collaboration is of course the huge interdependence of Mexico and the United States; Hispanics are now the largest minority in the United States, and Mexicans are the largest group within the Hispanic population. There is clearly a convergence, we recently had in Cancun the meeting of President Bush, President Fox, and Prime Minister Harper from Canada. There is a whole new initiative call—The Safety and Prosperity Initiative for North America—that has an explicit component of converging standards in regulatory frameworks, and we have clearly a movement towards greater convergence and I think we ought to take advantage of it.

The idea of a joint task force is very appealing, we have had a very good history of successfully initiatives between Mexico and the United States. One that has been extremely successful has been the Binational Health Weeks. I had the chance to talk during lunch, I know they had to leave, both, with Diana Bonta and Xochitl Castaneda, which have been very instrumental; in 2001 we have had a week in October, perfectly synchronized between Mexico and the United States for a great number of health promotion activities. Last year was the fourth year we have done Binational Health Weeks and it was present in 33 states of the United States, 33 Mexican states, and now it is even in two provinces of Canada as well. The Binational Health Week has become a great venue, it has been very successful, if we can do this joint task force that would be very good, and if a concrete product is to leave this national plan, in addition to the first steps that have been taken by this administration and previous administrations, can be carried forward, I think that would be very helpful.

Every road, even the longest road has a first step, we have to take that first step, and I think with the work that you have done in this past couple of days we are better equipped to look forward to that step. Health has the great virtue of being a unifying value. Even though sometimes we do not have a very comfortable relation with our neighbors, partners, and friends in the United States we have always found that health matters are a way of really bridging the two societies. I think this could be yet another successful example of binational collaboration if the IOM in the United States, which has had a great history of collaboration with Mexico particularly with its current president Harvey Fineberg, and this National Institute of Public Health here as a great center for analysis, reflection, research, data, can build this bridge and combine all the actors, certainly on the Mexican side, industry, NGOs, the other academic institutions. I think we could be on the path of taking very helpful measures for the Mexican population both here and in the United States and in that way pursuing the health of both countries.

Let me finish by thanking each and everyone, especially those of you who have traveled to come to Cuernavaca for this seminar. I can see from the wealth of conclusions that it has been a very fruitful time. I will do whatever I can do in the remaining seven months of this administration to support this work. Seven months is a lot of time, we can do a lot of things; no one in the Ministry of Health is packing, we do not feel like we are leaving, maybe it is a distorted self-perception, but we are feeling with the same energy as on day one; so you can be assured that the value of knowing that you have a deadline is that then the sense of urgency is even more pressing. We have seven months to deliver a high-quality product; let us take that first step on the long road. Thank you to everyone for having contributed to this joint enterprise.

REFERENCE

IOM (Institute of Medicine). 2005. *Preventing Childhood Obesity: Health in the Balance.* Washington, DC: The National Academies Press.

A

Workshop Agenda

Institute of Medicine
Joint U.S.–Mexico Workshop on Childhood Obesity Prevention

National Institute of Public Health of Mexico

Av. Universidad No. 655, Col. Santa Ma. Ahuacatitlán,
Cuernavaca, Morelos 62508
Phone: +52-777-329-3000 ext. 3371

Cuernavaca, Morelos

May 3–4, 2006

STATEMENT OF TASK

The IOM in collaboration with the National Institute of Public Health in Mexico will convene a two-day workshop to explore common issues and potential for collaboration in the area of preventing childhood obesity in populations of Mexican origin. From the perspective of the United States and Mexico, workshop presentations will consider the nature of the problem, current policies and programs to address it, lessons learned from current interventions, and potential public policy approaches.

AGENDA

Wednesday, May 3, 2006

9:00–10:00 am Moderators:	**OPENING SESSION** *Juan Rivera, Instituto Nacional de Salud Pública (INSP), Cuernavaca, Morelos* *Jeffrey Koplan, Emory University, Atlanta, GA*
9:00–9:30 am	**Welcome and Introduction to INSP** *Jaime Sepúlveda, Secretaria de Salud* *Mauricio Hernández, Instituto Nacional de Salud Pública*
9:30–9:45 am	**Welcome from Institute of Medicine/Food and Nutrition Board. Workshop Agenda and Goals** *Reynaldo Martorell, Emory University*
9:45–10:15 am	**Self Introduction of Participants** *Jeffrey Koplan, Emory University*
10:30 am–1:30 pm Moderator:	**PLENARY PRESENTATIONS** *Jeffrey Koplan, Emory University*
10:30–10:45 am	**Overview of IOM Childhood Obesity Prevention Report** *Jeffrey Koplan, Emory University*
10:45–11:10 am	**Group Discussion**
11:10–11:30 am	**BREAK**
11:30–11:50 am	**Preventing Obesity in Mexican-American Children and Adolescents** *Fernando Mendoza, Stanford University, CA* *Frederick Trowbridge, Trowbridge & Associates, Inc., Decatur, GA*

11:50 am–12:10 pm	**Preventing Obesity in Mexican Children and Adolescents** *Bernardo Hernández, Instituto Nacional de Salud Pública* *Ruy Lopez, Instituto Nacional de Salud Pública*
12:10–1:30 pm	**Group Discussion**
1:30–4:00 pm	**LUNCH**
3:00–4:30 pm	**WORKING GROUPS SESSION** **Working Group 1: Common themes/factors. Differences and similarities between United States and Mexico** **Working Group 2: Evidence gaps in data** **Working Group 3: Actions implemented. Opportunities, challenges, and barriers**
4:30 pm	**Adjourn for the Day**

Gala Dinner at 7:30 pm in Restaurant "El Madrigal"

Thursday, May 4, 2006

8:30–10:00 am Moderator:	**WORKING GROUPS SESSION** (cont.) *Esteban Cruz, Kaiser Permanente*
8:30– 9:00 am	**Working Groups Presentations** *Rapporteurs*
9:00–10:00 am	**Group Discussion**
10:00 am–1:30 pm Moderator:	**PLENARY SESSION: OPPORTUNITIES AND CHALLENGES** *Jaime Sepúlveda, Secretaria de Salud*

	PANEL PRESENTATIONS
10:00–11:00 am	**Panel 1: The roles of the public sector and private sector in preventing childhood obesity** • **Families and communities** • **Private sector** • **Public sector**
11:00–11:20 am	**BREAK**
11:20 am–12:20 pm	**Group Discussion**
12:20–12:40 pm	**Panel 2: Opportunities for collaboration: A bi-national, common agenda to prevent childhood obesity**
12:40–1:45 pm	**Group Discussion**
1:45–3:00 pm	**LUNCH**
3:00–3:30 pm	**SUMMARY AND CLOSING REMARKS** *Juan Rivera, Instituto Nacional de Salud Pública* *Julio Frenk, Secretaria de Salud*
3:30 pm	**Adjourn**

B

Preventing Obesity in Mexican Children and Adolescents

Ruy López Ridaura, Research Center for Population Health: Chronic Disease Division, Instituto Nacional de Salud Pública (National Institute of Health, INSP)
Simón Barquera, Research Center for Nutrition and Health, INSP
Bernardo Hernández Prado, Research Center for Population Health: Reproductive Health Division, INSP
Juan Rivera, Research Center for Nutrition and Health, INSP

INTRODUCTION

Mexico is among many countries that have experienced a rapid increase over the past two decades in the proportion of children and adolescents with excessive weight. In the decade between the First (1988) and Second (1999) National Nutrition Surveys, there was an increase in the prevalence of Mexican children ages 2–4 years who were either obese or at risk for obesity,[1] rising from 21.9 percent to 28.7 percent. This is the only age group in children for which national trend data are available. For older Mexican children, the lack of national trend data limits the evaluation of obesity trends during that decade. However, data from the Second National Nutrition Survey show equally alarming evidence of a growing obesity epidemic in children and youth. Based on the age- and gender-specific body mass index (BMI) charts developed by the Centers for Disease Control and Prevention (CDC) in 2000 (Kuczmarski et al., 2000), 21.1 percent of Mexican children ages 6–11 years have a BMI equal to or greater than the 85th percentile and are considered to be obese (8.8 percent) or at risk for obesity (12.3 percent). Among girls ages 12–19 years, 22.3 percent have a BMI

[1]At risk for obesity and obesity are defined as having a BMI equal to or greater than the 85th and 95th percentiles, respectively, of the age- and gender-specific BMI charts developed by the CDC in 2000 (Kuczmarski et al., 2000).

equal to or greater than the 85th percentile and are either obese (5.7 percent) or at risk for obesity (16.6 percent).

These data reflect an evolving obesity epidemic, representing an enormous burden for the public health and health care systems in Mexico. The association between childhood obesity and many health risks, in both children and adults, has been consistently found. The major public health impact is the association of childhood obesity with chronic disease risks in adulthood, especially overweight and obesity, type 2 diabetes, hypertension, asthma, hyperlipidemia, cardiovascular diseases (CVD), and certain cancers. Excessive weight at younger ages has also been associated with adverse psychosocial outcomes such as low self-esteem, depression, anxiety, and impaired cognitive function, especially in adolescents, although findings have not always been consistent (Swallen et al., 2005). However, research is currently not available to demonstrate this association in Mexican children and youth.

Nutrition-related chronic diseases represent a serious public health problem for the Mexican population. According to the Organization for Economic Cooperation and Development (OECD) 2005 Health Report, one quarter (24.2 percent) of the Mexican adult population is classified as obese (OECD, 2005). Data from the most recent National Health Survey (2000) showed that nearly 8 percent of all Mexican adults over 20 years of age have type 2 diabetes and approximately 30 percent have hypertension (Olaiz et al., 2003). Moreover, type 2 diabetes and CVD are the leading causes of death in the adult Mexican population, and some small studies suggest an increasing incidence of type 2 diabetes and glucose intolerance at younger ages (Cruz et al., 2004; Rodríguez-Moran et al., 2004).

Although there has not been a comprehensive evaluation of the economic impact of obesity in Mexico, a recent analysis estimated an attributable cost of diabetes for the public health sector of approximately $317 million U.S. dollars for the year 2005, almost equally distributed between direct and indirect costs (Arredondo and Zuñiga, 2004). The increasing incidence of obesity at younger ages and the scarce public resources in the country will considerably aggravate these economic projections.

As in many developing countries, the Mexican population is in the process of an epidemiologic transition and is experiencing a double disease burden. Child mortality rates and the incidence of infectious diseases have decreased. However, statistics show a significant increase in obesity and related chronic diseases such as diabetes, hypertension, and CVD in adults. High rates of malnutrition and related problems are still observed, especially among sub-populations of Mexican children. This paradoxical situation is the result of multiple factors, partly attributed to the uneven development among different segments of the population and increased socioeconomic inequalities (Uauy et al., 2001). A closely related phenomenon that the Mexican population has experienced over the past few decades is a nutritional transition, that is a shift in the overall structure of dietary patterns and a reduction in energy expenditure. This transition is affecting most of the population, and has been proposed that it is the main driving force of the obesity epidemic and related chronic conditions in developing countries (Popkin, 2001).

Given the concern over the growing prevalence of obesity and its impact, the U.S. Congress directed the CDC in 2002 to request that the Institute of Medicine (IOM) develop an action plan targeted to prevent obesity in U.S. children and youth. The IOM convened a multidisciplinary committee to develop a prevention-focused action plan. In 2004, the committee released the report *Preventing Childhood Obesity: Health in the Balance* (IOM, 2005), which proposed a set of recommendations for a variety of sectors and stakeholders that, when implemented together, would catalyze synergistic actions to effectively prevent the large majority of children and youth in the United States from becoming obese and facilitate the adoption of healthier lifestyles. By making childhood obesity a national priority, this set of recommendations calls on coordinated actions among the government, industry, media, community organizations, schools, and families that together will develop a broad-based public health strategy needed to effectively halt and decrease this growing epidemic (IOM, 2005).

Are these recommendations applicable to Mexican–American and Mexican children and youth? Are these recommendations applicable to the particular public health challenges faced by Mexico? Is there any benefit to developing a common binational obesity prevention agenda or strategy? These are the main questions that stimulated the IOM to sponsor a joint U.S.–Mexico workshop—in collaboration with the National Institute of Public Health in Mexico (INSP) and supported by Kaiser Permanente—that will focus on exploring a binational approach to obesity prevention and the adaptation of the IOM report recommendations to Mexican children and youth living in the United States and in Mexico. The purpose of this paper is to review the factors that contribute to obesity in Mexican children and adolescents, provide an overview of current programs addressing this problem, and propose a set of actions that may offer the greatest potential for success in preventing and controlling the epidemic. A companion paper, authored by U.S. colleagues, will address obesity trends and determinants in Mexican–American children and youth (Trowbridge and Mendoza, 2007) and provide a complementary view to the issues presented in this paper.

Based on an ecologic perspective, several components and their degrees of influence are context specific. For instance, the acceptance and understanding of "healthy behavior" recommendations are linked closely to cultural values that could be specific for each ethnic group. Also, given that most of the recommendations imply actions at different normative levels, there are substantial differences in the legal, economic, and political contexts that need to be considered carefully in the use of the IOM report model to develop recommendations for Mexican children and youth living on both sides of the U.S.–Mexico border.

Approaching obesity prevention among Mexican children and youth as a binational problem could have many advantages. Given the strong link between the population in Mexico and the one that has migrated to the United States, common cultural perceptions and values can be explored as a combined effort to design culturally acceptable recommendations and to define research priorities. Moreover, the permanent relationship, including remittances and transfer of commodities between U.S. migrant workers and their families, might allow the development of coordinated strategies that could impact not only the population living at the border (characterized by a high mobilization across countries) but also the population living in the remote areas (especially the rural areas) of Mexico, where most migrants trace their family roots. Finally, the obesity burden, on one hand, and the evidence of effective programs in the United States, on the other, can potentially improve advocacy efforts in Mexico and vice versa. Therefore, if coordination between countries can be fostered, progress toward effective preventive interventions will be accelerated with benefits and impacts on both sides of the U.S.–Mexico border.

DEFINING THE PROBLEM

Definition and Measurement of Obesity

BMI, which is calculated by dividing weight in kilograms by height in squared meters (kg/m^2), is a useful indirect measurement of body fat and unhealthy weight in children ages 2 years and older and adults. It is often used as a screening tool to identify individuals who are obese and those at risk for obesity because the measurements of height and weight are easily obtained compared with skinfold thickness measurements and other complex procedures that require more training and standardization. BMI is one of the best indicators of body fat, which is proposed as the cause component of the health consequences associated with obesity (Mei et al., 2002). Indeed, BMI has been associated consistently with several risk factors, even among children and adolescents. Preliminary results of the association between BMI and chronic disease risk factors among Mexican adolescents based on the National Health Survey (2000) are consistent with analyses from other countries in which CVD risk factors show a dose–response relationship with BMI categories, whereby the normal-weight category shows the lowest risk profile and the obesity category shows the highest risk pro-

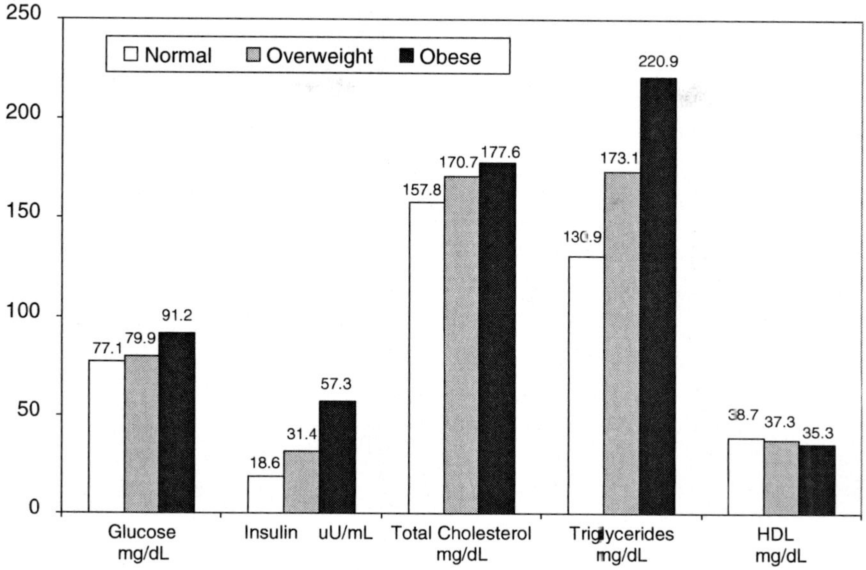

FIGURE B-1 BMI categories and their association to CVD risk factors in children and adolescents ages 10–19 years, from the Mexican Health Survey (2000).
SOURCE: Villalpando et al. (in press).

file (Villalpando et al., in press) (Figure B-1). BMI has certain disadvantages. It has been suggested that other indicators, such as waist circumference, waist-to-hip ratio, or skinfold thickness measurements, could have a stronger association with metabolic abnormalities. However, these measurements are not usually obtained for children and youth in health clinics and school systems as readily as weight and height, and are usually not known by parents; thus, BMI is the measurement most commonly used.

Although there may be a need to develop ethnic-specific definitions for overweight and obesity, the cut-off points used to define overweight (a BMI between 25 and 29.9 kg/m^2) and obesity (a BMI equal to or greater that 30 kg/m^2) for adults are widely accepted. However, given that BMI changes with children's growth and development, it is more appropriate to use age- and gender-specific BMI charts to define obesity and at risk for obesity in children and adolescents. For consistency with the IOM report *Preventing Childhood Obesity: Health in the Balance* (IOM, 2005) and with the companion paper examining the factors contributing to obesity in Mexican–American children and youth, this paper uses the CDC BMI charts established in 2000 to define obesity and being at-risk for obesity for children and adolescents between the ages of 2–19 years. According to this reference, children and adolescents with a BMI equal to or greater than the 95th percentile are considered obese, and those with a BMI between the 85th and 95th percentiles are considered to be at risk for obesity (IOM, 2005; Kuczmarski et al., 2000). In the absence of a reference population or cut-off points specific for the Mexican population, the authors conclude that the CDC BMI charts are the best available for children and adolescents 2–19 years. In the future, the recently released WHO Child Growth Standards, developed using data collected by the World Health Organization (WHO) Multicentre Growth Reference Study that provide new guidelines for assessing obesity in children ages 0–5 years (WHO, 2006a) could also be used for that age range.

Obesity Prevalence and Trends in Children and Youth in Mexico

The only national survey that included anthropometric measurements of school-aged children was the Second National Nutrition Survey (Rivera et al., 2001), conducted by the National Institute of Public Health of Mexico between October 1998 and March 1999. The Third National Nutrition Survey 2006 is currently in progress and will provide further data on obesity trends in children, youth, and adults throughout the entire country.

The results of the Second National Nutrition Survey were based on a national probabilistic sample of 17,944 households. The sampling methodology and response rates are described in detail elsewhere (Resano-Pérez et al., 2003). The resulting sample is representative at the national level of urban (≥ 2,500 people) and rural (< 2,500 people) sites and of four geographic regions: north (the wealthiest region), south (the poorest region), Mexico City [a large urban center with the greatest socioeconomic status (SES) contrasts], and central (including states that are generally between the north and the south with respect to SES). The study population included children younger than 5 years of age (n = 8,011), school-aged children ages 5–11 years (n = 11,415), and women ages 12–49 years (n = 18,311). The sample represented about 10.6 million children 4 years of age or younger and 15.6 million children ages 5–11 years. In addition to these age ranges, which were employed in the First and Second Mexican National Nutrition Survey and are used in previous publications, for consistency with the IOM report (IOM, 2005) and the companion paper on Mexican–American children, we computed prevalences for the following age ranges (Table B-1): 0–23 months, 2–5 years, 6–11 years, and 12–19 years. However, some of the results presented in this document use the age ranges employed by the National Nutrition Surveys because we obtained them from published material.

The national prevalence of children at risk for obesity and obese by age, geographic region, and sociodemographic characteristics derived from the National Nutrition Survey 1999 are illustrated in Table B-1. In infants younger than 2 years, the national prevalence of children at risk for obesity [defined as the percent > +2 SD of the WHO/National Center for Health Statistics (NCHS)/CDC reference population] is 5.84 percent. For children ages 2–5 years, the prevalence of obesity (BMI ≥ 95th percentile of the age- and gender-specific CDC BMI charts) was 10.4 percent, and the prevalence of children at risk for obesity (BMI between the 85th and 95th percentile of the CDC BMI charts) was 17.1 percent for a total of 27.5 percent of children in this age category who are either at risk or obese. Both groups present higher prevalence in the north compared with the other regions, and for 2–5-year-olds, the prevalence was higher in urban versus rural areas and in high versus low SES strata.

The only age category for which there are available data from two national surveys (1988 and 1999), allowing for an evaluation of obesity trends, is children younger than 5 years of age. Figure B-2 shows the trend in the proportion of children ages 2–4 years that were over the 85th percentile of the reference population. An increase was evident at the national level (31 percent, from 21.9 percent to 28.7 percent) and in each of the four regions represented in the survey; this increase was especially notable in the north (with the highest SES), which showed an estimated increase over 50 percent (from 20.8 percent to 31.8 percent) in the prevalence of obesity or at risk for obesity (> 85th percentile) over the 11-year period. This increment was mainly driven by the proportion of children who were at risk for obesity rather than the obesity category.

Among Mexican children ages 6–11 years, 8.8 percent were classified as obese (> 95th percentile) and 12.3 percent were classified as at risk for obesity (> 85th percentile) at the national level. The magnitude of the regional prevalence followed the children's SES status. The highest prevalence of obesity was found in the north (12.7 percent), followed by Mexico City (11.4 percent), the central region (8.8 percent), and the south (5.5 percent). The prevalence was higher in those living in urban (11 percent) versus rural areas (3.4 percent), in children whose mothers had a higher level of formal education (e.g., more than high school = 13.2 percent, high school = 11.8 percent, primary school = 7.5 percent, without formal education = 4.8 percent), and in the non-indigenous population (9.4 percent versus 3.4 percent). The prevalence of children at risk of obesity was higher than for the obesity category following the same pattern. The relatively larger prevalence of unhealthy weight in wealthier subpopulations is in contrast with the very small differences in prevalence of unhealthy weight found among the same subpopulations for adult women (Rivera et al., 2002).

TABLE B-1 Prevalence of Children at Risk for Obesity and Obese by Age and Selected Geographic and Socio-Demographic Characteristics

	0–23 months	2–5 years		6–11 years		12–19 years	
Age category	Wt-for-ht (WHO)	Age- and gender-specific BMI charts (Kuczmarski et al., 2000)					
Indicator		At Risk	Obese	At Risk	Obese	At Risk	Obese
Cut-off points	> +2 SD	85–95	> 95	85–95	> 95	85–95	> 95
National	5.84	17.1	10.4	12.3	8.8	16.6	5.7
Region							
North	7.1	19.5	12	15.5	12.7	18.3	10.1
Center	4.6	17.7	9	11.6	8.8	17.4	7
Mexico City	5.7	13.6	9.7	15.5	11.4	20.7	3.8
South	6.3	16.7	11.3	9.6	5.5	13.4	3.2
Location							
Rural	5.6	17.1	10.8	8.6	3.4	12.8	4.2
Urban	6.4	17.2	9.8	13.9	11	18.2	6.3

Gender							
Girls	6.7	18	9.7	12.1	8.5	16.6	5.7
Boys	5	16.3	11.1	12.4	9.1	-	-
Maternal education							
More than high school	7.2	19.3	12.1	14.2	13.2	-	-
High school	6.8	16	10.3	15.7	11.8	-	-
Elementary school	4.4	17.4	9.6	11.6	7.5	-	-
No education	5.4	15	8	8.7	4.8	-	-
Socioeconomic status							
High	5.5	17	11.7	15.4	14.1	19.2	7.7
Medium	6.1	16.2	11.6	14.4	10.5	16.4	7
Low	6.2	17.8	8.6	7.3	2.4	14	2.2
Indigenous ethnicity							
No	5.9	17.0	10.6	12.5	9.4	16.7	5.9
Yes	5.2	18.6	9.1	9.9	3.4	15.8	3.2

NOTES: Results from the 1999 Mexican Nutrition Survey. All prevalence is expressed as a percentage considering sampling weights. Definitions for obesity and at risk for obesity use the 85th and 95th age- and gender-specific percentiles from the 2000 CDC BMI charts for all age categories except children ages 0–23 months that were defined using > 2 SD of weight for height from the WHO/NCHS/CDC reference population. For the age category 12–19 years, data are exclusively for women.
SOURCE: Rivera et al. (2001).

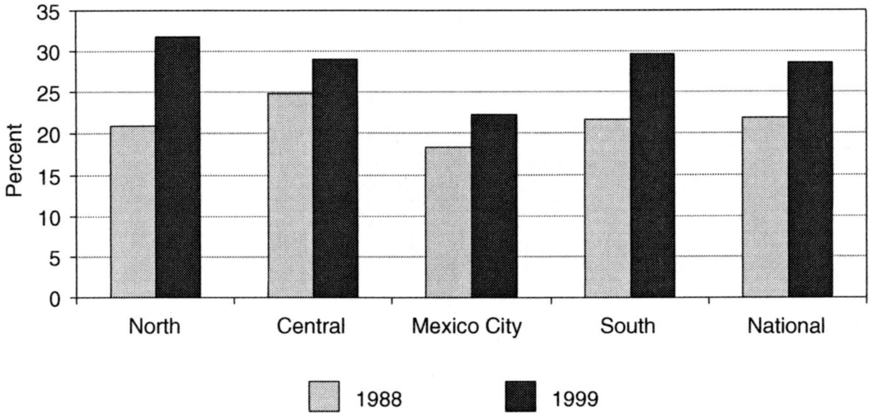

FIGURE B-2 Prevalence of risk of obesity or at risk for obesity by region and year of survey (children ages 2–4 years).
SOURCE: Rivera et al. (2001).

Undernutrition and Catch-Up Growth in Children and Youth in Mexico

The coexistence of under- and overnutrition is a characteristic of the Mexican population, particularly among children and young women. Along with the high prevalence of unhealthy weight in children, the prevalence of stunting,[2] anemia, and micronutrient deficiencies remain public health concerns. Stunting continues to be an important public health problem in children younger than 5 years of age while wasting[3] is no longer a widespread problem, decreasing from a national prevalence of 6 percent in 1988 to a prevalence of 2 percent in 1999. At the national level, stunting occurred in almost one of every five children younger than 5 years of age (17.7 percent) while wasting occurred in only 2 percent. The mean height-for-age z-score in this age group was -0.8 ± 1.3 while the mean weight-for-height z-score was $+0.2 \pm 1.1$. Stunting occurs predominantly during the first two years of life. The prevalence increases almost threefold between the first and the second years of life (from about 8 percent to 22 percent) and remains at about 20 percent up to 4 years of age. From 5–11 years, the percent of

[2]Stunting is defined as low height for age (< 2 SD of the WHO/NCHS/CDC reference population).

[3]Wasting is defined as low weight for age (< 2 SD of the WHO/NCHS/CDC reference population).

stunting in children was 16.1 percent, which is mainly the result of stunting during early childhood. The long-term effects of stunting on height are evident in the adult population. On average, Mexican adult women are short (e.g., the mean height of women 12–49 years of age is 152.9 cm).

Anemia and micronutrient deficiencies are widespread in most age groups (Villalpando et al., 2003a, b, c). More than one in every four children younger than 5 years (27.2 percent) are anemic, and between one-quarter to one-half have one or more micronutrient deficiencies. The prevalence of iron, zinc, and vitamin A deficiencies are at approximately 52 percent, 33 percent, and 27 percent, respectively. Additionally, more than 25 percent of children have serum ascorbic acid concentrations indicative of low dietary intake of vitamin C. Some micronutrient deficiencies occur predominantly at younger ages. Anemia rates peak in the second year of life, when almost half of all children are affected, but decrease to about 17 percent prevalence at 4 years of age. Iron deficiency affects about two-thirds of all children between 1 and 2 years of age and less than 50 percent between 3 and 4 years of age.

The prevalence of anemia in children ages 5–11 years was 19.5 percent; it was slightly higher in rural (21.9 percent) than urban (18.3 percent) areas, higher in indigenous (24 percent) than non-indigenous (18 percent) children, and much lower in Mexico City (11 percent) than in other regions (18 percent to 24 percent). The micronutrient with the highest deficiency prevalence was iron (36 percent), followed by vitamin C (30 percent), vitamin A and zinc (about 20 percent), and folic acid (about 10 percent). Urban areas had a much lower prevalence of iron and zinc deficiencies (38.2 percent and 18.2 percent, respectively) than rural areas (48.3 percent and 40 percent, respectively) (Rivera and Sepúlveda-Amor, 2003).

As mentioned earlier, stunting is a public health problem in Mexico, but the prevalence of wasting is within expected values for a healthy population. Results from the Second National Nutrition Survey (Rivera et al., 2001) show that the mean height-for-age z-score is –0.4 from 0–11 months, drops to –1.1 at 12–23 months, and remains at around –1.0 up to 59 months of age. The prevalence of stunting is 8.5 percent from 0–11 months of age, rises sharply to 21.8 percent at 12–23 months, and remains at about that level until 4 years of age. These data indicate that stunting occurs from birth to 23 months of age and that there is no substantial catch-up growth from 23 to 59 months. At the end of the preschool period, the height of children is about 1 SD below the mean value of the reference population, and about 20 percent of children have heights in the lower extreme (< –2 SD) of the reference distribution. In contrast, the mean weight-for-height z-score remains between +0.1 and +0.3 from birth to 59 months of age, indicating that weight relative to height is slightly above the value expected given the height of the population. Moreover, wasting remains below 3.5 percent from birth to 59 months.

For older children important catch-up growth is not observed either, especially in low socioeconomic conditions. Data from the Second National Nutrition Survey 1999 showed that children ages 2–9 years from the upper 25 percent of the SES index have higher values of height-for-age relative to the rest of the population (average differences 3.8 cm in girls and 4.1 cm in boys) but are still shorter than the WHO/NCHS/CDC reference (average differences 1.6 cm in girls and 1.8 cm in boys) (Figures B-3 and B-4) (Monterrubio-Flores, 2006). Thus, whereas the prevalence of stunting for 5–11-year-old children is about 16 percent, the prevalence of BMI > 85th percentile of the 2000 CDC BMI charts in this age category ranges from 19 percent to 35 percent (average = 25.7 percent) in boys and from 21 percent to 43 percent (average = 28.6 percent) in girls (Rivera et al., 2001). This contrast indicates that even though linear catch-up growth is not achieved, weight relative to height, i.e., BMI, is high.

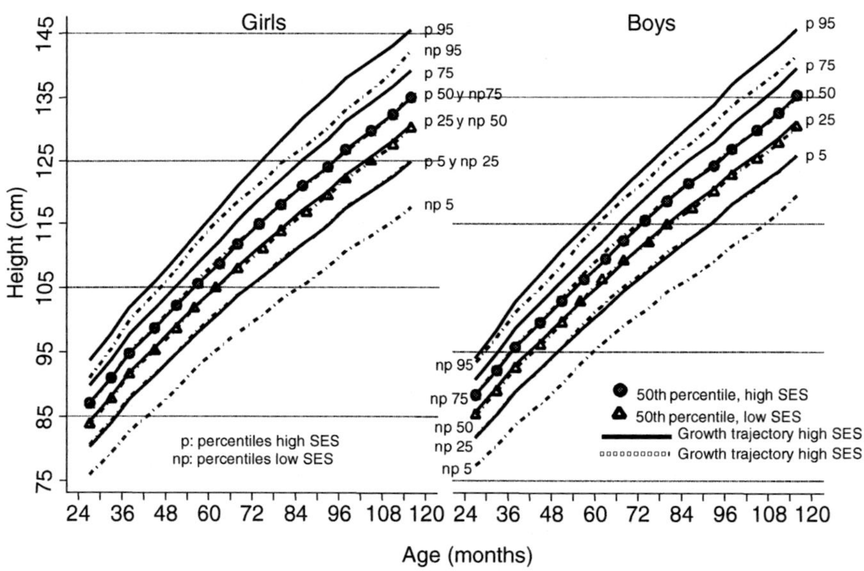

FIGURE B-3 Height-for-age calculated percentiles for Mexican children ages 2–9 years old, according to socioeconomic status (SES).
NOTES: Calculated percentiles are based on the entire Mexican population. SES is classified by the SES index distribution using the 75th percentile as the cutoff point—high is > 75 percent and low is < 75 percent.
SOURCE: Monterrubio-Flores (2006).

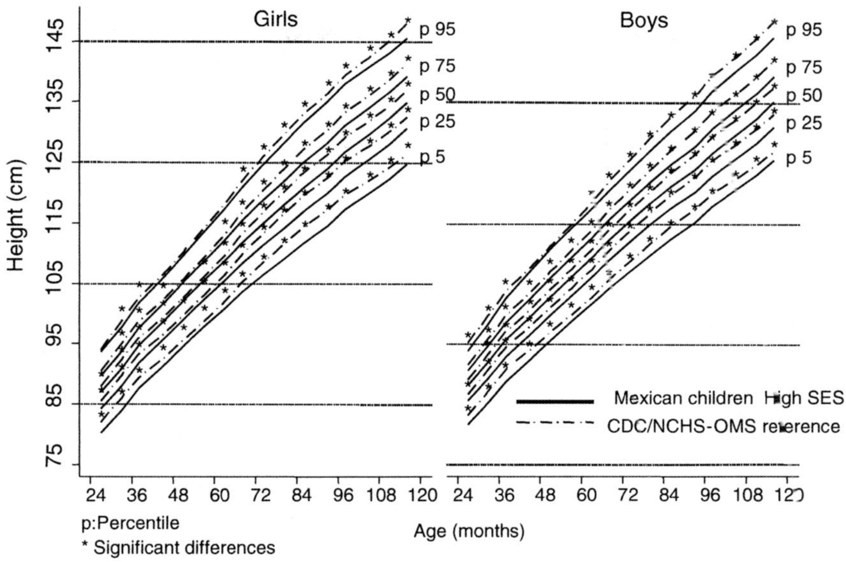

FIGURE B-4 Height-for-age calculated percentiles for Mexican children ages 2–9 years from the upper quartile of socioeconomic status (SES) distribution versus the CDC/NCHS-OMS reference population.
NOTES: Calculated percentiles are based on the entire Mexican population. SES is classified by the SES index distribution using the 75th percentile as the cutoff point. high is > 75 percent and low is < 75 percent.
SOURCE: Monterrubio-Flores (2006).

The aforementioned data show that childhood obesity represents a growing problem in Mexican society, a problem that will add an additional burden to a health care system already preoccupied and overwhelmed by public health issues related to poverty and underdevelopment. When comparing prevalence of under- and overnutrition in the populations of the United States and Mexico, two important differences emerge. First, the Mexican data clearly reflect a dual burden—the problem of undernutrition (especially stunting) and micronutrient deficiencies are unsolved and therefore require ongoing public health strategies and monitoring systems for addressing the problem. In contrast, these problems are not widespread in the American population and thus are not public health priorities. Second, the prevalence of childhood obesity in Mexico is higher among wealthier groups, whereas in the United States, the populations at greatest risk for obesity are ethnic minorities (e.g., African Americans, Hispanic Americans, American Indians) and lower SES families. Interestingly, this latter difference does not occur in the Mexican adult population, in which obesity is much more homogeneous among SES groups. This difference in the distribution of obesity among SES groups between children and adults may be related to low SES households providing environments that are more prone to encourage infections and malnutrition, especially among young children. These differences should be considered when formulating recommendations to prevent obesity in children and adolescents in Mexicans living in Mexico and those living in the United States.

FACTORS INFLUENCING CHILDHOOD AND ADOLESCENT OBESITY

In order to define a set of recommendations for preventing obesity among Mexican children and youth, the relative contribution of different determinants driving the problem must be examined. Although several scientific observations have built strong evidence on the biological and socioeconomic determinants of obesity, the relative contribution of these factors is context specific. This section contains an analysis and description, based on the best available evidence, of the relative weight of potential determinants in the Mexican context.

Using an ecologic framework to understand the determinants of obesity, it is clear that several factors at different levels interact to explain energy imbalance, which is the direct cause of obesity. The next section reviews the relative contribution of the two main factors related to energy balance—energy intake versus energy expenditure—and explores the social and cultural factors influencing them in the Mexican context. The authors use available evidence to describe how the environment has changed for Mexican children and youth over the last few decades toward an "obesogenic" environment, understood as an environment that may promote obesity and encourage the expression of an individual's predisposition to gain weight.

Energy Balance and Individual Factors

Obesity can be viewed as a problem of a positive energy balance—in other words, an excess energy intake relative to a given energy expenditure sustained over time. Even a minor energy imbalance over time can result in the accumulation of excess body fat. During childhood and adolescence, adequate balance should be kept in order to allow normal growth. When energy intake exceeds expenditures, including the requirement for normal growth and development, then body fat accumulates and the risk of obesity increases. Dietary intake represents the energy intake side of the energy balance equation, while energy expenditure has several components—resting metabolic rate, adaptive thermogenesis, the thermogenic effect of food, and physical activity (Horton, 1983).

In addition to energy intake, other factors, including genetics, can explain the variability between populations in linear growth. However, there is consensus that the variability in linear growth across regions is due more to social, demographic, and economic factors than to genetics, at least among preschool children (Habicht et al., 1974). In an international comparison using the WHO global database on child growth and a database of national factors, Frongillo et al. (1997) concluded that most national variability of stunting and wasting among preschool children was explained by national factors and geographic region where higher energy availability, female literacy, and gross product were the most important associated factors. The genetic contribution to linear growth after puberty remains unknown.

In the last few decades, extensive research has focused on the search for a genetic component in the etiology of obesity, and consequently some evidence on the role of genes in the obesity etiology has been documented (Snyder et al., 2004; Chagnon et al., 2000; Oksanen et al., 1997; Rosenbaum and Leibel, 1998). According to the "thrifty genotype" hypothesis, originally proposed in the sixties by James Neel (1962), Indian ancestry could be a genetic risk factor for metabolic syndrome features, including obesity; the hypothesis could partially explain the individual predisposition observed in highly admixed populations such as Mexicans. An analysis among Mexican Americans in San Antonio, Texas, showed that diabetes risk augments as the Native-American admixture increases estimated from skin color measurements (Gardner et al., 1984). Recently, the use of ancestral indicator markers has been proposed as an alternative methodology to evaluate this hypothesis and for genetic mapping purposes, although its effectiveness remains to be proven (Fernandez and Shiver, 2004). However, for the moment there has not been a gene or even a unique genomic region associated consistently with obesity risk. More importantly, the fact that the observed worldwide trends in obesity cannot be explained by modification on the genetic pool of populations suggests a minor role of the genetic component in the current obesity epidemic. Moreover, as a nonmodifiable factor, the contribution of genetic factors in designing effective obesity preventive strategies may have a minor role when compared to environmental and behavioral factors.

Another proposed factor that may increase individual susceptibility to obesity and related chronic diseases such as CVD and diabetes, other than genetic susceptibility, is malnutrition in early life, especially low birth weight (LBW) and stunting before the age of 3 years (Caballero, 2001). The increasing prevalence of noncommunicable chronic diseases affecting more people at younger ages in developing countries than in the developed world (WHO, 2006b) may suggest an extra vulnerability of populations in epidemiologic transition, such as the Mexican people. If nutritional insults in early life confer this extra vulnerability, then the results of combating undernutrition in early life (gestation and the first 2–3 years of life) will have double benefits—adequate nutritional policies will affect not only the undernutrition-related problem but also the increasing epidemic of chronic diseases.

After observing an association of LBW and low height at 1 year of age with hypertension and other CVD, Barker (1992) proposed the fetal origin of disease hypothesis, later known as thrifty phenotype hypothesis, as an alternative to the thrifty genotype hypothesis previously described (Hales and Barker, 2001). This hypothesis (called "programming hypothesis") suggests that poor fetal or early life nutrition causes an adaptation process that increases the capacity to store energy, and thus may program future propensity to obesity, diabetes, and CVD. Since then, several studies (mainly in developed countries) have tried to test this hypothesis with inconclusive results. The association between LBW or short stature during early life and the risk for diabetes and hypertension has been observed in several populations (Simmons, 2005). However, other studies have failed to observe the same association (Stern et al., 2000; Lucas et al., 1999). The size of the effect and its relative impact of the programming hypothesis on the high prevalence of these diseases in developing countries remain controversial.

In terms of the risk of developing obesity in adulthood, the impact of fetal or postnatal growth retardation remains unclear. Large cohort studies such as the Nurses' Health Study have shown a J-shape in the association of birth weight and adult obesity, with both LBW as well as high birth weight showing an increased risk relative to normal birth weight (5.6–7 pounds, equivalent to 2.5–3.8 kg) (Rich-Edwards et al., 1999). The impact of postnatal growth retardation on the risk of obesity is less clear. For instance, the study—which because of its natural design has been recognized as quasi-experimental—of records on the Dutch famine during World War II has shown that the prevalence of adult obesity was higher among those exposed to famine during the first two trimesters of pregnancy than among those exposed during the last trimester and early infancy. This last group had an even lower prevalence of obesity than those who were not exposed to the famine (Stein et al., 1995).

One of the reasons for the inconsistency of the results may be the fact that the majority of these studies have been performed in developed countries, where there is a low prevalence of undernutrition and therefore the effect could be low. On the other hand, the majority of these studies have shown that LBW and stunting are not risk factors per se. The increased risk may be expressed only among subjects who move from a scarcity to an abundance of energy intake. Studies characterized by their nutritional transition with clear modifications in dietary patterns and lifestyle are needed from developing countries to support or reject this hypothesis. However, analysis of a Guatemalan population showed that fetal programming might have a minor role at least for CVD risk among adults (Stein et al., 2002.)

Although the programming hypothesis is still controversial, while new evidence from developing countries arises the potential contribution of LBW and short stature during the first years of life in the definition of preventive strategies should be considered, especially in Mexico where stunting remains as a prevalent problem. In contrast to the genetic component information, the basis of programming theory could be modified in just one generation if researchers succeed in controlling undernutrition during early life. This implies investing in nutrition promotion programs in early life as a potential strategy for obesity prevention.

Levels of Physical Activity and Inactivity

Although there is limited information on levels and trends of time dedicated to physical activity and inactivity in Mexican children and youth, the available information indicates a tendency to sedentary lifestyles. In a study conducted on children and youth ages 9–16 years in low- and middle-income schools in the Mexico City area, they devoted an average of 4.1 hours/day to total video viewing (representing total leisure screen time except computer use) and only 1.8 hours/day to moderate or vigorous physical activity. Boys reported more television viewing and time spent in physical activity than girls (Figure B-5) (Hernandez et al., 1999).

Another study conducted using a similar methodology with youth and young adults ages 11–24 years in the state of Morelos, Mexico, found results that also suggest a sedentary lifestyle. In this case, adolescent boys and young men reported significantly more time dedicated to moderate and vigorous physical activities than girls and young women. Boys spent more time playing videogames [3.2 (SD 2.4) hours daily], than watching television [2.7 (SD 1.9) hours daily], while adolescent girls and young women spent 2.6 (SD 2.5) hours daily using VCR or videogames and 2.8 (SD 1.9) hours daily watching television. Significant differences in the mean daily screen time—defined as total hours per day watching television, videogames, or VCR—were observed by age, type of community, SES, and medical insurance in both adolescent boys and girls and young adult men and women. Adolescent girls who reported that they were dieting to lose weight had significantly less screen time exposure than girls who wanted to gain weight. Mean screen time significantly increased with the level of urbanization of the community, and, in girls and young women, screen time increased with

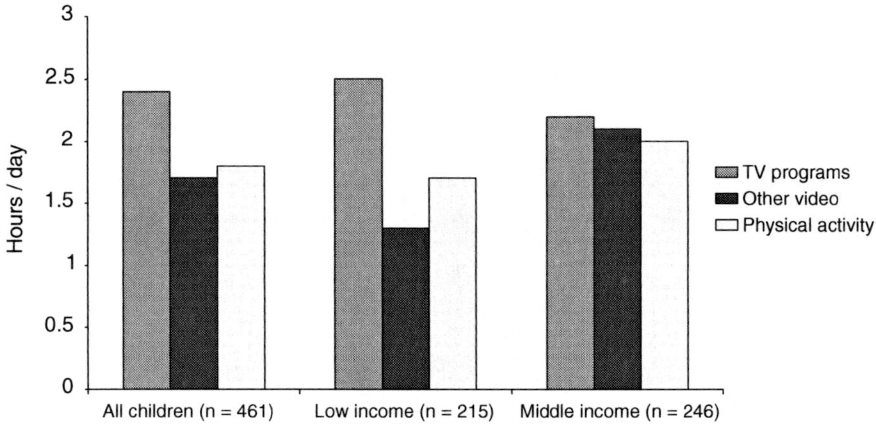

FIGURE B-5 Mean time dedicated to video viewing and physical activity, Mexico City children and youth ages 9–16 years, 1999.
SOURCE: Hernandez et al. (1999).

increasing SES ($p < 0.01$) (Lajous M; personal communication; August 2004; Cancun, Mexico). A study using data from the Second National Nutrition Survey (1999) found that adolescent girls and women ages 12–49 years dedicated an average of 45 minutes/day to physically active sports and 3.64 hours/day to television viewing. Thirty-four percent of the adolescent girls and young women ages 12–20 years old reported that they practiced sports regularly, and they had higher odds of practicing sports than women ages 31–49 years old (Hernandez et al., 2003).

The association between television viewing and obesity (as measured by BMI levels) has been documented (Gortmaker et al., 1996; Robinson, 2001). This association also was found in Mexico in the studies mentioned previously. In the study conducted with children in Mexico City, after adjustments for other covariates such as parental obesity, SES, age, and gender, children who spent more than 3.1 hours/day viewing television programs were 1.69 times more likely to be obese or at risk for obesity than children who viewed television programs less than 1 hour/day. On the other hand, children who engaged in physical activity less than 1 hour/day were 1.6 times more likely to be obese or at risk for obesity than children who engaged in physical activity more than 2.5 hours/day. When analyzing the associations between television program viewing, physical activity, and being obese or at risk for obesity, similar associations were found (Table B-2) (Hernandez et al., 1999). There were related findings in the study conducted with youth in the state of Morelos in which a BMI of 0.13 kg/m^2 higher (95 percent CI 0.04, 0.23) was found in adolescent boys who spent

TABLE B-2 Adjusted Odds Ratios for Children Ages 9–16 Years at Risk for Obesity and Obese by Television Program Viewing and Physical Activity Level, Mexico City, 1999

VARIABLE	Odd Ratios	Confidence Interval 95%
Television programs (hours/day)	1.12	(1.02, 1.22)
Moderate/vigorous physical activity (> 3 Mets/hour) (hours/day)	0.90	(0.83, 0.98)
Vigorous physical activity (> 6 Mets/hour) (hours/day)	0.80	(0.70, 0.92)

NOTE: Adjusted by age, gender, zone of residence, and mother's perception of figure. Mets= metabolic equivalents for task.

more than 5 hours/day viewing television compared with adolescents who viewed television less than 2 hours/day ((Lajous M; personal communication; August 2004; Cancun, Mexico).

Eating Pattern Trends: Nutritional Transition

As stated previously, Mexico is experiencing a nutritional transition with a clear shift over the past decades to higher intakes of fat, refined carbohydrates and processed foods, and lower intakes of whole grains, vegetables, and dietary fiber that represent traditional diets (Popkin, 2001; Rivera et al., 2004a). The transition is closely related to the process of urbanization and the migration from rural areas into the cities but also is affecting the rural areas to a lesser extent. The relationship among the nutritional transition, urbanization, and poverty is complex and manifests differently in various countries. Studies have shown that the nutritional transition was observed mainly among the higher SES groups living in rural areas and among low SES groups in urban areas, suggesting that lower-income populations, principally in urbanized environments, could be affected by the two extremes of the nutritional spectrum (Seidell, 2000). In Mexico, the nutritional transition, as assessed by changes in dietary fat intakes and BMI values in adults, has been observed in all regions regardless of their level of development, in urban and rural areas, and in all socioeconomic groups. In contrast, as presented previously, high BMIs in children are more prevalent in the more developed regions and urban areas. However, evidence suggests that children living in low-income neighborhoods and attending public schools in Tijuana along the Mexican side of the U.S.–Mexican border are

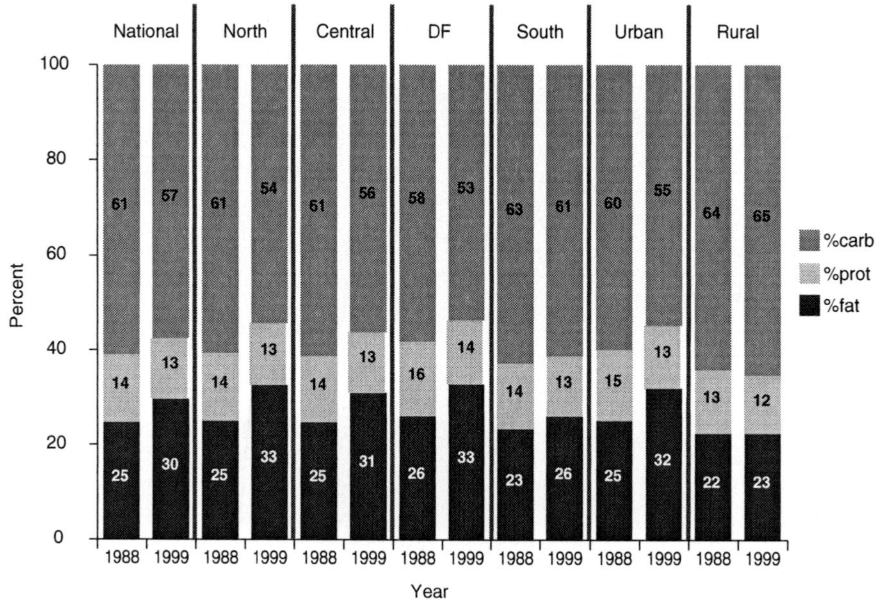

FIGURE B-6 Relative contribution of macronutrients to total energy intake from 1988 to 1999.
SOURCE: Barquera et al. (in press).

experiencing a nutrition transition with respect to an increased risk of obesity and related chronic disease (Villa-Caballero et al., 2005).

The strongest evidence of this transition comes from the contrast between adults' self-reported dietary intakes from the 1988 and 1999 National Nutritional Surveys. During this 11-year period, the percentage of energy intake from fat among Mexicans increased from 23.5 percent to 30.3 percent (Figure B-6). This increment was observed across all regions of the country, including the poorest region (south), which increased from 22.1–26.9 percent during the same time period (Rivera et al., 2004a). However, this increment was not observed in rural areas, where the percentage of energy intake from fat remained stable at 22–23 percent. Unfortunately, there is a lack of information about changes in the type of fats (e.g., saturated, trans fat, and unsaturated fat) in the Mexican diet, especially for children and youth.

In this same analysis, the mean percentage of energy intake from carbohydrates decreased slightly from 59.7 percent to 57.5 percent. However, the lack of information on the type of carbohydrate (especially in the 1988 survey) limits the possibility to analyze intakes of refined versus complex

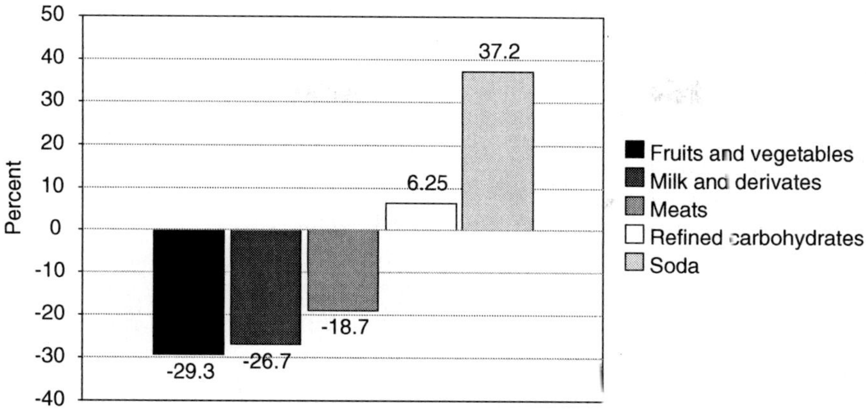

FIGURE B-7 Changes in mean food purchases in 1996 (relative to 1994) by food group.
SOURCE: Rivera et al. (2004a).

carbohydrates. A secondary analysis using data from National Income and Expenditure Surveys collected by the Instituto Nacional de Estadística, Geografía e Informática (INEGI) from 1984 to 1998 showed that consumer purchases of refined carbohydrates and sweetened sodas increased by 6.3 percent and 37.2 percent from 1984 to 1998, respectively, whereas the amount of fruit and vegetables purchased dropped by almost 30 percent during the same period (Figure B-7) (Rivera et al., 2004). This observation suggests that complex carbohydrate intake has declined. Whether or not the modification of relative prices of these food commodities during this period played an influential role in the consumer purchases is an area that requires further research.

In the Second National Nutrition Survey 1999, dietary intake for school-aged children was evaluated using a 24-hour dietary recall. Foods were ranked according to their contribution to the total amount of food intake (in grams). Four food groups represented nearly 50 percent of their total amount of food consumed. The main contributors to children's diets were milk and dairy products (185.5 g), tortilla and maize products (156.4 g), and sugar and sugar-sweetened beverages (135.3 g). Only 8 percent of the children had fruits and vegetable intakes greater than 400 g/day, which represents the current recommended intake (WCRF, 1997), while 56 percent had intakes less than 100 g/day (Figure B-8) (Ramirez CI and Rivera JA; personal communication; February 2006). The median energy intake in preschool children was 949 calories and 1,377 in school-aged children. Pro-

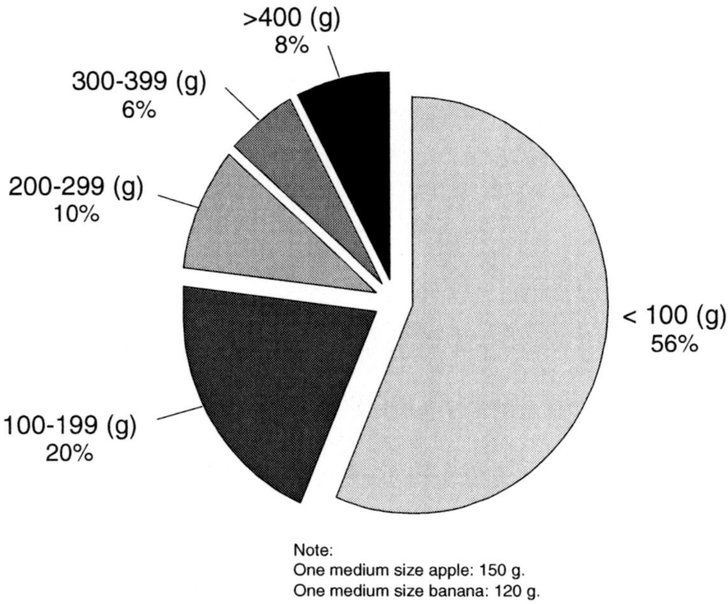

FIGURE B-8 Distribution of school children according to fruit and vegetable consumption based on the Second National Nutrition Survey, 1999.
SOURCE: Barquera et al. (2003).

tein intake in both groups was well above adequate levels at 150 percent of estimated requirements. Children living in the northern and Mexico City regions had the highest fat intake and the lowest fiber intake. Children living in the southern region, indigenous children, and those in the lowest SES group had higher fiber and carbohydrate intakes and the lowest fat intake (Barquera et al., 2003).

A study conducted using data from the Second National Nutrition Survey 1999 classified foods consumed by children ages 1–4 years as either centrally processed or not processed. Centrally processed foods are defined as those involving any kind of industrial process, whether they are foods that had been consumed without industrial process before (e.g., milk or bread) or foods that were developed by industry (e.g., sweetened soda and packaged snack foods). Centrally processed foods made an important contribution to the total energy and nutrient intakes at the national level and in sub-populations. For example, the contribution to total energy intake was 46 percent; protein intake was 39 percent; total fat intake was 56 percent; and saturated fat intake was 69 percent. These findings underscore the im-

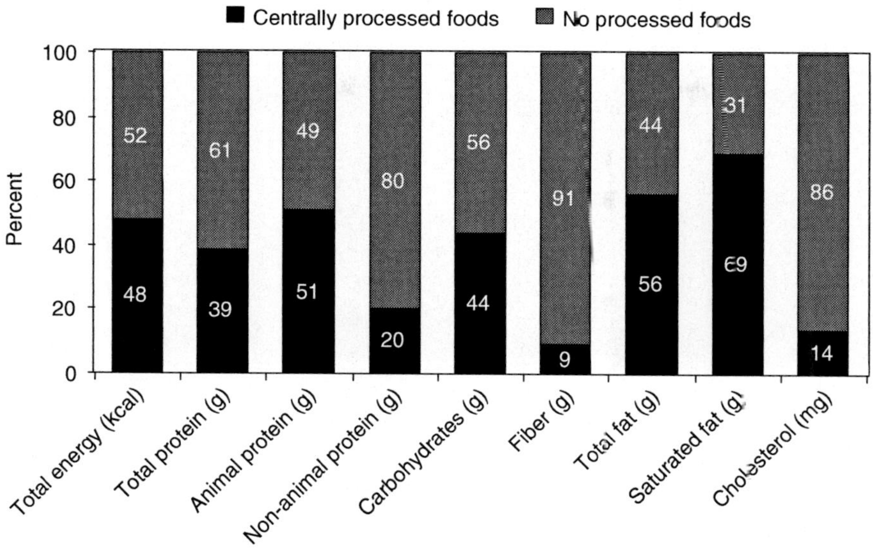

FIGURE B-9 Contribution of centrally processed foods to total energy and nutrient intakes in children younger than 5 years old.
SOURCE: González-Castell et al. (2003).

portance of the food and beverage industry in the diets of preschool children and demonstrate the need for involving food and beverage companies in efforts to prevent and control childhood obesity (González-Castell et al., 2003) (Figures B-9 and B-10).

Factors that Influence Energy Intake and Energy Expenditure

Family and Sociocultural Factors

Family and cultural values are strong determinants of both eating patterns and physical activity levels (Patrick and Nicklas, 2005). Although direct evidence was not available on the role of family and cultural values as determinants of childhood obesity in Mexico, there is anecdotal evidence suggesting that chubby children are perceived to be healthy children, especially among the poorest and rural sub-populations, in Mexican society. Researchers are unaware of any empirical evidence supporting this widespread cultural belief or its origin. It has been suggested that recent and concurrent undernutrition in the same communities or even in the same families, reinforce the ideas that heavier children are healthier. In a small

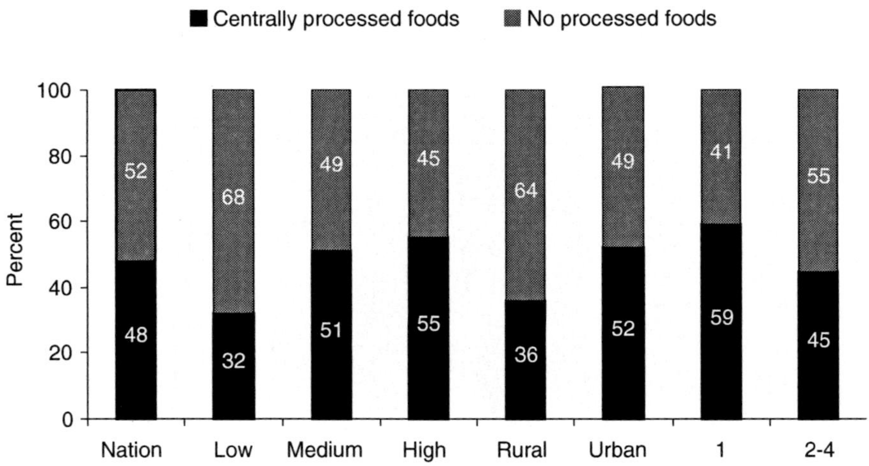

FIGURE B-10 Contribution of centrally processed foods to total energy intake of population subgroups (nationwide, low socioeconomic status (SES), medium SES, high SES, rural, urban) in children younger than 5 years old and 1 or 2-4 years old.
SOURCE: González-Castell et al. (2003).

study in Xalapa, Veracruz, half of all parents of obese children did not identify their own children as having any weight problem (Brewis, 2003). This parental perception suggests either a level of denial or a normalization of obesity that reinforces children to be heavier than the accepted healthy range. These beliefs, combined with other cultural values such as feeding a child as an act of love and caring, or that acquiring and using consumer goods that decrease physical activity such as television, video games, and cars are identified as markers of higher SES within communities, need to be counterbalanced with community-based interventions that empower parents and key community members to promote healthier lifestyles. This is an area where both observational and experimental research are greatly needed.

Self-reported energy intake can vary considerably between non-obese and obese subjects. Based on data from the Second National Nutrition Survey 1999, researchers estimated energy under-reporting in Mexican women ages 18–49 years using a 24-hour dietary recall questionnaire. Researchers found that the prevalence of energy under-reporting in non-obese women was approximately one-third (33.66 percent) and more than half (53.73 percent) in obese women. The adjusted prevalence ratio for under-reporting was 1.51 times higher in obese compared with non-obese women (95 percent CI 1.35, 1.69). The researchers concluded that obese Mexican women tend to under-report energy consumption more than their non-obese counterparts. The differential under-reporting in Mexico between obese and non-obese women suggests that there is a perception of the association between diet and excess weight, which may be a positive sign of increasing awareness of the epidemic (Campirano et al., 2003). However, experimental studies in children and adolescents have shown that mean daily caloric intakes may be under-reported by as much as 17 to 33 percent of energy expenditure and that under-reporting tends to increase with age (Bandini et al., 2003; Champagne et al., 1998). Similar methodological challenges exist for conducting research on children's physical activity levels (IOM, 2005).

Another factor that may influence dietary patterns and physical activity is the change in family structure experienced in Mexico during the last two to three decades. The following additional issues also may influence dietary and physical activity patterns: the increase of women's roles in the labor force, increasing rates of divorce and single parenthood, increasing numbers of families with key members in the United States, and decreasing household size. For example, reduced time available for food selection and for cooking can encourage the use of more energy-dense processed food and therefore can influence the quality of the diet. Also, reduced time of parents at home coupled with increasing levels of insecurity in the streets may encourage television viewing and sedentary lifestyles. However, empirical evidence of these possible effects in Mexico is lacking.

Environmental Factors: Transition Toward an Obesogenic Environment

Opportunities for physical activity. Information about access and use of television and the Internet indicates that Mexico is moving toward a more sedentary environment. The number of television stations operating in the country has increased from 115 in 1980 to 658 in 2004 (Secretaría de Comunicaciones y Transportes, 2005). Not surprisingly, by 2000 85 percent of the households in Mexico had access to a television set, and this proportion reached 97 percent in Mexico City. Even in the states with a high poverty level, such as Chiapas or Oaxaca, more than 56 percent of the households had a television set (INEGI, 2000). Mexico has a higher number of television sets per capita than most Latin American countries, although the number is still lower than that in the United States (Figure B-11). However, exposure to television in Mexico can be underestimated because Mexican households are larger than those in the United States. Restricted television (television systems that charge for access) also is becoming more popular, increasing from 1,250,000 subscriptions in 1995 to 2,660,000 in 2003 (COFETEL, 2005).

In addition to the explosive growth of the television industry in Mexico, the Internet also is becoming more popular. The number of Internet users grew from 94,000 in 1995 to 16,492,454 in 2005 (INEGI, 2005a). Most

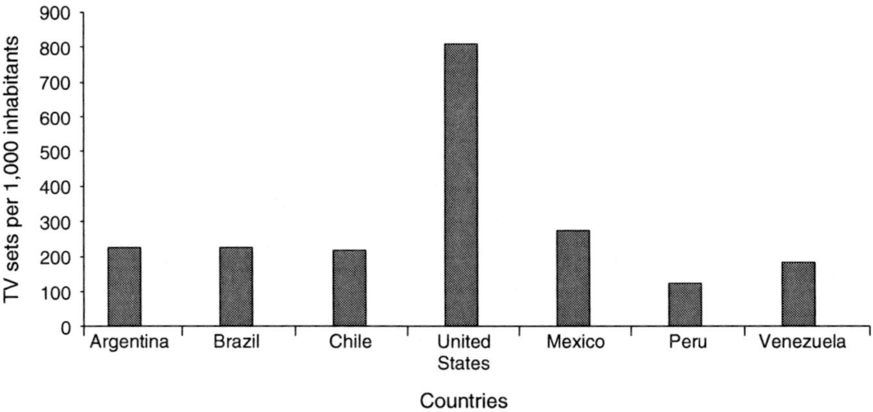

FIGURE B-11 Number of television sets per 1,000 inhabitants, selected countries, 1997.
SOURCE: COFETEL (2005).

importantly, Internet use is concentrated in youth and adolescents, as shown in Figure B-12, rising from 2.43 percent to 7.73 percent between 2001 and 2005 for children ages 6–11 years and from 14.41 percent to 34.16 percent between the same years in adolescents ages 12–17 years. Finally, it is estimated that more than 22.8 million Mexicans—13.1 percent of 6- to 11-year-old children and 28.1 percent of 12- to 17-year-old adolescents—use computers (INEGI, 2005b).

Another indicator suggesting that the Mexican population is moving toward an obesogenic environment with reduced options to engage in physical activity is the growth in the number of motorized vehicles. Although the population of Mexico has increased 17 percent from 1990 to 2000, the number of motor vehicles registered increased by 38 percent during the same period of time, representing nearly 11 million automobiles in 2000 and 13.5 million automobiles in 2002 (INEGI, 2005b).

Trends in access to unhealthy and healthy foods. Over the past few decades, Mexicans have experienced an increased availability and access to less healthful foods and beverages (e.g., high energy–dense, low nutrient–dense, and low-fiber foods and high-calorie low-nutrient beverages). This is especially true for Mexicans living in urban areas. This increased access to these types of foods and beverages is yet another fact indicating the country is shifting toward an obesogenic environment.

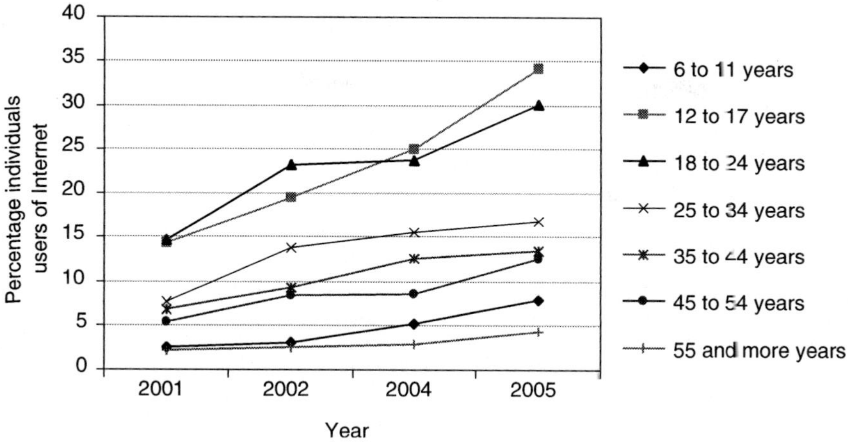

FIGURE B-12 Percentage of Mexicans who are Internet users by age group, 2001–2005.
SOURCE: INEGI (2005b).

Transnational corporations representing the fast food restaurant or quick serve restaurant industry have expanded substantially over all the major and middle-size cities across Mexico. The first Mexican franchise of McDonald's Corporation opened in 1985 in one of the wealthiest neighborhoods of Mexico City. According to the company's website, there are currently 320 franchises nationwide located not only in wealthy areas but also in middle- and low-income neighborhoods (McDonald's Corporation, 2006). A very similar phenomenon has happened with other restaurant companies such ALSEA, which operates Domino's Pizza and Burger King in Mexico. According to a company report (ALSEA, 2005), over 15 years, the quick serve restaurant company has established 529 Domino's Pizza sites in 123 cities and promoted sales of more than 37 million pizzas in 2004. Indeed, hamburgers and pizza are the major types of fast food restaurants representing 30 percent and 37 percent, respectively, of the entire fast food market in Mexico. The success of these companies relies on the acceptance of their products by Mexicans. Given the huge consumer demand, the meals are affordable for a large proportion of the population (Hawkes, 2002).

Another form of energy-dense foods that are widely available is Mexican street foods that are sold informally on the streets in cities as well as in schools. Although data are limited about the numbers of sites, varieties, prices, and nutrient-content of the Mexican street foods, this industry appears to be rooted in Mexican culinary culture and its growth has paralleled the population growth in urban areas. An important feature of this industry is the modification of traditional Mexican food that usually was not fried and contained tomato, hot pepper, and other vegetables. However, current street foods sold are high energy–dense as a result of widespread use of vegetable oil for frying, increasing the use of cream and cheese, and reducing the use of vegetables. Therefore, this "Mexican fast food," which is not centrally processed, is an important source of total energy in the Mexican diet, including children and youth.

As with the fast food restaurant industry, the high consumption of sweetened beverages, particularly carbonated soft drinks, in Mexico is linked to large-scale marketing activities across multiple media platforms (e.g., print, radio, broadcast and cable television, Internet, outdoor signage). Indeed, according to a WHO report that reviewed marketing activities of global soft drink and fast food companies in emerging markets, Mexico was identified as the world's leading per-capita consumer of Coca-Cola. In 1998, Mexicans consumed more than 400 milliliters per day of sweetened carbonated soft drinks. By volume of sales, Mexico is the Coca-Cola Company's second largest market after the United States (Hawkes et al., 2002).

Another important source of energy in the Mexican diet is the high intake of oil. The use of oils with a high *trans* fatty acid content has increased considerably in both the fast food industry and in baked and fried foods and snacks produced by industry. Also, high fructose corn syrup has been replacing the sugar cane as a sweetener in soft drink production, although some evidence exists about its potential impact on weight gain (Bray et al., 2004), this is still a topic of much debate. The association of certain types of fats or sweeteners to obesity remains unknown and needs further research.

Advertising and marketing trends. In 2004, food advertising was ranked fourth and beverage advertising was ranked sixth in 20 categories for the amount spent on advertising to Mexicans through television, radio, and print media totaling US $1.064 billion and US $565 million, respectively. Television advertising is the primary venue for food and beverage advertising to the Mexican population (WARC, 2005). There were limited data publicly available to the authors documenting the growing trend of companies' promotion of high energy–dense and low nutrient–dense foods and sweetened beverages, sedentary activities, and entertainment to Mexican children and youth. There are data showing that fast food restaurant and beverage companies engage in philanthropic activities and sponsorship of sporting events as ways to market to Mexican youth (Hawkes, 2002). The Global Kids Study, conducted in 1996 and 1998 by Just Kid Inc., Nickelodeon, and Research International, provides information about the brand and consumer environment, attitudes, beliefs, and consumption behaviors of a cohort of 400 children, ages 7–12 years, and their mothers who were surveyed in each of six countries. The purpose of the marketing research was to provide Nickelodeon with a strategic planning tool to support the entertainment company's international business initiatives targeting children and youth in countries such as Mexico. The cities where the study was conducted in Mexico include Mexico City, Guadalajara, and Monterey. An interview and questionnaire were used to gather detailed marketing research data about the children and their families. The findings showed that international global brands, such as Coca-Cola, McDonald's, Pizza Hut, and Kentucky Fried Chicken, are well recognized by Mexican children based on their brand awareness and preferences (Friend and Stapylton-Smith, 1999). There are presently no publicly available data documenting Mexican children's and youths' discretionary income, particularly among higher SES groups, which they may use to purchase foods and beverages without parental guidance, especially away from home settings such as fast food restaurants, shopping malls, and schools.

Consumers ages 18 years and younger are subject to special protection under Mexican law. However, there is currently no single governmental authority or body of law governing products or advertising to Mexican children and youth. The three government institutions primarily responsible for the regulation of children's advertising in Mexico are the Attorney General for Consumer Protection, Ministry of the Interior, and the Ministry of Health (Arochi et al., 2004). The non-governmental self-regulatory organization in Mexico is the National Council for Advertising (Consejo Nacional de la Publicidad) (Friedman and Dickler, 2003). There are clear guidelines and laws restricting the promotion of alcohol and tobacco products to Mexican children. According to Article 16 of the Communications Council Code of Ethics, advertisers must not "undermine parental authority, judgment, or preferences" and "children should not be encouraged to urge other persons to purchase a product, especially their parents." Companies are also encouraged to avoid taking advantage of children's credulity or lack of experience. While television and radio advertising should not exceed 18 percent of the total time of transmission to Mexicans, special regulations for children's advertising have not yet been developed in Mexico. Furthermore, there are currently no guidelines or regulations for the promotion of high-calorie and low-nutrient foods and beverages to young consumers (Arochi et al., 2004).

However, Mexico is one of the many countries that endorsed the WHO Global Strategy on Diet, Physical Activity, and Health at the 57th World Health Assembly in 2004 (WHO, 2004). The Global Strategy provides member states with a range of policy options to address less healthful dietary practices and physical inactivity, including provisions for marketing, advertising, sponsorship, and promotion to support international public health goals. These provisions recommended that "food and beverage advertisements should not exploit children's inexperience or credulity," should discourage messages that promote less healthful dietary practices, and encourage positive healthful messages (WHO, 2004).

School environments. Unhealthy weight in children, particularly in school-age children, results from an environment that enhances the intake of high energy–dense foods and restricts the opportunities for regular physical activity. Children spend a substantial amount of time at school. Therefore, the school environment is an important influence on their physical activity behaviors and dietary patterns.

The Ministry of Education implements a physical education program in elementary schools nationwide (Secretaría de Educación Pública, 1994) that envisions two physical education sessions, each lasting about 30–50 minutes per week, as a means to promote a healthy lifestyle. The program also aims to promote a healthy diet through elementary-level educational materials that include units related to hygiene and nutrition and the promotion of healthful lifestyles.

The physical education component of the program is structured according to the different skills and development characteristics attributable to each age group. The program is designed to promote five different types of skills. Stimulation of motor perception; conditional physical skills; basic sports skills building; physical education for health; and social interaction. The plan includes a section that suggests several activities and one more that recommends methods for evaluating the plan's performance. Nevertheless, the program is not implemented as designed according to existing policies.

Researchers conducted a search for publications on the school environment and its relationship to childhood obesity in Mexican schools but was not able to find published articles on this topic. However, formative research was obtained from a project that was recently initiated in 12 public schools in Mexico City; the project aims to change the core elements in the school environment that promote obesity (Rivera J, National Institute of Public Health; personal communication; March 2006). The first phase of the project undertook an assessment of the school environment. Preliminary data from children in 4th and 5th grades in 12 schools representing over 1700 students showed that children, are exposed to an unhealthy environment in several ways. Children are exposed to high energy–dense foods (e.g., high-fat and high-sugar snacks and foods such as candy, ice cream, pizza, pork skin chips with cream, tacos, and other traditional Mexican fried foods) and to large portion sizes. In addition, children eat several times at school (they have as much as six feeding opportunities during the four hours at school). The availability of fresh fruits and vegetables is very limited, and most often the available fruits are served with cream. The preparation and handling of foods sold in schools are under uncertain sanitary conditions that increases the food safety risks for the children. Additionally, most of the schools lack free drinking water from fountains. In the few schools where potable water fountains are available, they are not well maintained and are not used for drinking water.

Physical activity is low. The school-break period is the time designed to eat lunch, and there is limited time left for active play or physical activity. During this time children are not allowed to run due to safety concerns, because all grades have recess at the same time and older children running or playing could harm younger children. In addition, there is limited space available for physical activity in many of the schools surveyed. In general, the school facilities and sports equipment do not facilitate adequate physical education classes and children spend on average less than 40 minutes of Physical Education (PE) per week, about 40 percent of the time established by norms (100 minutes per week). Moreover, PE classes are not active enough; children spend only nine minutes per week on moderate to vigorous physical activity.

These results are similar to findings from a small pilot study in 10 schools in Mexico City. In this sample, approximately half of the schools in the pilot study did not have appropriate areas for the physical education classes; the average space available was 290 m^2 for approximately 330 students. Moreover, teachers showed little motivation to promote physical activity, and the physical education classes were not well structured. Approximately 30 percent of children did not participate in physical education classes, and moderate to vigorous physical activity was achieved for approximately 10 minutes by those participating in the physical education classes. In 80 percent of the schools the average length of the physical education class is 50 minutes a day, and the remaining 20 percent of the schools divide the class length by age groups (30 minutes for children younger than 10 years of age and 50 minutes for older children) two times per week. Only 20 percent of the schools organize and promote extracurricular sporting events such as soccer and athletics tournaments. One of the major limitations of extracurricular physical activity programs is that many schools have several shifts (e.g., morning and evening) at the same facility, so that extracurricular physical activity programs are not possible. The following issues were identified as potentially important in terms of their influence on behavior and dietary intake at school:

- Lack of drinking water from water fountains or other public supplies at schools in seven of the eight schools surveyed, which may promote the intake of sweetened beverages.

- Lack of bottled water and the widespread availability of sweetened beverages in concession stands that have similar prices; therefore, there may be a reduced incentive for the children to drink water during the school day.
- Lack of regulations for foods and beverages sold either at concession stands on the school grounds or at retail establishments located near schools.
- The federally funded and mandatory school breakfast program provides energy-dense and centrally processed foods at very affordable prices.
- Widespread availability of high energy–dense foods and sweetened beverages within and around the school environment.
- Low availability of vegetables and fruits within and around the school environment.

Although this formative research is not representative of public schools throughout Mexico, or even the schools in Mexico City, it provides a qualitative assessment of the school environment that may be useful to identify the elements within the environment that promote obesity and opportunities for positively intervening to promote a healthier school environment.

Other environmental factors. These factors are important determinants of an environment favoring a positive energy balance in most of the Mexican population. However, there are many other factors that are likely to influence children and youth and can be considered components of an obesogenic environment. However, there is limited research on these factors upon which to design evidence-based strategies for effectively preventing obesity in Mexican children and youth.

The exponential growth of mega cities in Mexico, with a lack of environmental design planning to facilitate physical activity, are likely to have an important impact on the availability and access to physical activity facilities, especially in poor and new neighborhoods in the suburbs of these cities. Data regarding availability and use of physical activity facilities are clearly needed to evaluate and potentially modify this factor. Another issue potentially contributing to reduced physical activity are safety concerns and poor air quality in Mexican cities, especially in Mexico City, which has been identified as one of the cities worldwide with the highest level of air pollution (Villarreal-Calderón et al., 2002).

Finally, with regard to energy intake, it is likely that a change in agricultural and food production policies favoring large-scale production, marketing supports for commercial producers, and developing a more competitive agricultural sector for export markets (Zahniser et al., 2005) could modify the price and access of certain foods but not necessarily the most healthful choices. Many of these policies adhere to international trade agreements such as North American Free Trade Agreement (NAFTA) (Zahniser et al., 2005); thus the impact and consequences they may have on the dietary patterns of the Mexican population has not been fully explored. Further research in this area is needed.

CURRENT POLICIES AND PROGRAMS

Despite the strong evidence of an increasing obesity epidemic among children and adolescents in Mexico, its impact on the awareness of the population at different levels has been limited. Within the last few years, perhaps as a consequence of published research and dissemination of the Second National Nutritional Survey 1999 results, the obesity epidemic has reached the media, especially print- and web-based media. Among the scientific community, obesity, particularly in children, is currently a topic that has generated a great deal of attention in terms of funding and human resources, with support for several ongoing research projects. However, there is still an enormous need for raising awareness at the individual, family, and community levels, as well as within the government sector at all levels. Probably because of the recent and still current problem of undernutrition as one of the main public health problems among children, the complete understanding of the double burden of undernutrition and obesity from the government and policymakers is needed to elevate childhood obesity as a national priority.

As a consequence of the low awareness within the government sector, there are a limited number of programs, mostly on a small scale, and information about these programs is not readily available. The next section describes selected programs and policies that are related to the obesity problem.

Government Policies on Food Labeling, Media Control, and Dietary Guidelines

Mexico has a set of policies, norms, and guidelines for food labeling and media control of advertising food products. However, there are many inconsistencies during the implementation of these policies, and many of them have not been periodically reviewed or modified in response to the increasing public health problem of obesity. There has not been any evaluation on consumer understanding and the impact of the information provided on food labels. Regarding the media control, as noted earlier, television advertising is the primary venue for food and beverage advertising to the Mexican population (WARC, 2005). However, there is a lack of data on the effects of advertising on Mexican children's preferences, purchase requests, and influence on household purchases of food and beverage products. Limited evidence indicates that there may be a rise in television advertising of processed foods and beverages high in sugar or fat, or both, and

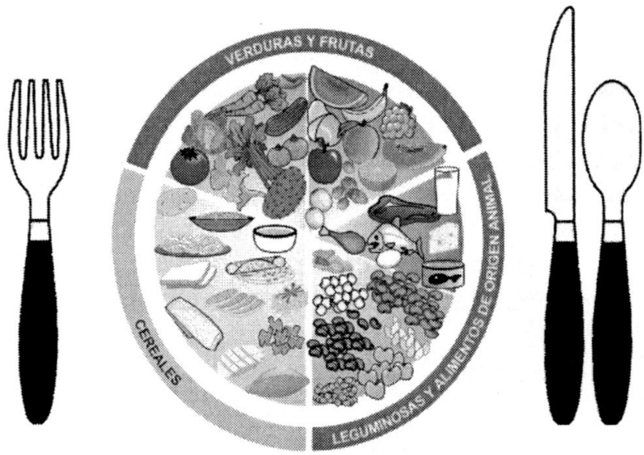

FIGURE B-13 El Plato del Bien Comer. Dietary guidelines.
SOURCE: Norma Oficial Mexicana (2005).

with healthy nutrition claims without specific policies guiding the health claims or types of advertising reaching young children.

For several years a group of nutrition experts has been working on developing dietary guidelines for Mexico. After a long process that led to consensus-based guidelines, they are soon to be officially published for the Mexican population. The guidelines are based on a plate model rather than a food guide pyramid (Figure B-13) and present food groups and advice on ways that consumers can combine them. Since these are consensus-based guidelines, this educational tool can be used as the basis for developing an effective communication strategy aimed at improving dietary practices in Mexico.

Social Programs

Oportunidades

The pillar of the Mexican social assistance strategy is the conditional cash transfer program, *Oportunidades*. The objective of the program is to break the intergenerational cycle of poverty though the development of human capital. At present, the program reaches more than five million families (about 25 million people) living in extreme poverty.

Oportunidades provides families with a monetary transfer intended for food purchase, a fortified food supplement for all children from 6 to 23 months of age, children aged 2 to 4 years with low weight for age, and for pregnant and lactating women; and educational scholarships conditioned on regular attendance in school, the size of which is grade and gender dependent. All benefits are conditioned on the use of regular preventative health services, the content of which changes over the life-course and regular attendance of the female head of household (to whom the monetary transfer is also given) to a series of health and nutrition education workshops. The program also provides curative health care (SEDESOL, 2006).

A number of positive impacts of the *Oportunidades* program on nutritional status of the population have been reported. In both urban (Neufeld et al., 2006) and rural Mexico (Rivera et al., 2004b) participation is the program resulted in an increase of approximately 1 cm in linear growth of children who were in the program from a very young age (< 6 mo) compared to children of similar age not in the program. A positive impact on the prevalence of anemia has also been reported among children less than 2 years of age (Rivera et al., 2004; Neufeld et al., 2005). However, there is concern that participation in the program may promote undesirable excess weight gain. Increased weight gain with improved socioeconomic status and higher income has been documented in a number of settings around the world (Uauy et al., 2001; Du et al., 2004). The extra resources provided to the family may be used to purchase more high energy–dense foods and sweetened beverages. The fortified food supplement for women and children provide approximately 1.4 and 2.15 kcal/g, respectively. In this population where the diet does not appear to have an energy deficit, regular consumption of the supplement in addition to the usual home diet without substitution of a similar quantity of energy may result in excess weight gain. Regular consumption is clearly desirable due to its high micronutrient content, approximately 100 percent of the Recommended Dietary Intake (IOM, 2001) of iron, zinc, and a number of other micronutrients known to be deficient in the diets of Mexican children and women during pregnancy and lactation (Rivera et al., 2003) . Consumption of the supplement has been shown to result in considerable improvements in the dietary intake of micronutrients and there is some indication of improvements in mineral status of women and children (Neufeld et al., 2006). On the other hand, the health and nutrition workshops and increased exposure to preventative health care services may lead to improved dietary and lifestyle choices among beneficiaries with a resultant decrease in the prevalence and/or severity of obesity.

The prevalence of obesity in adults who were eventually enrolled in the program (before program benefits were received) was over 20 percent (Fernald et al., 2004). In women living in urban Mexico, program participation was associated with a greater increase in body mass index over a two-year follow-up period compared to non-participants, particularly among those who had high body mass index at the start of the follow-up

(Neufeld et al., 2006). There was an increase of 1.5 percent in the prevalence of obesity in adolescents involved in the program when compared to adolescents who did not participate (Gutiérrez et al., 2005). Among preschool children, there is no evidence that participation in the program is associated with obesity, although there was a tendency towards higher BMI among the children who were enrolled in the program before 6 months of age, compared to non-beneficiaries (Neufeld et al., 2006).

The *Oportunidades* program with its system of co-responsibilities and its broad coverage is a promising vehicle through which to launch obesity prevention. Two studies are currently underway as part of the program evaluation activities to further clarify the impact of the program on weight gain among women and children and to strengthen the health education component of the program in reference to obesity prevention. The first is a large randomized controlled trial implemented within the context of the program. The main objective of the study is to determine whether regular consumption of the fortified food supplement is associated with increased weight gain among children and women during pregnancy and increased weight retention post partum compared to two other supplements with identical micronutrient content but without additional energy. The second study uses qualitative research methods to gain an understanding of the perceived determinants of overweight and obesity in the population and barriers to change in behaviors associated with excess weight gain. The results of both studies will be presented to decision makers within the program with specific recommendations of how to strengthen obesity prevention among program beneficiaries.

Health-Sector Programs

Preven-IMSS

The National Institute for Social Security (IMSS) provides health services to approximately 50 percent of the Mexican population. As part of the organization's process of health improvement services, they recently designed and implemented an integrated health programs strategy known as *Preven-IMSS*. This strategy is focused on a portfolio of preventive actions aimed at improving the health status of their target population and marks the first time that IMSS has launched a large-scale prevention program. Starting in 2002, actions were organized by age group and vulnerable populations: children (younger than 10 years of age), adolescents (ages 10–19 years), women (ages 20–59 years), men (ages 20–59 years), and older adults (older than 60 years of age). All the programs include major food and nutrition, physical activity, and health education components (Gutiérrez-Trujillo, 2005).

The main preventive actions for children are focused on health promotion, nutrition education, disease control and prevention, early identification of diseases, oral health, vaccination, and miscellaneous actions (e.g., personal hygiene, breastfeeding promotion, and fever control). For adolescents, the program's preventive actions are focused on physical activity promotion; accident prevention; violence and addiction prevention; oral health; sexual health and education; nutrition education; obesity detection and control; parasite treatment; vaccination; use of preservatives; human immunodeficiency virus and sexually transmitted diseases prevention; visual, auditory, and postural defects; and reproductive health. There are also components for adults.

For each preventive action, there is a set of designed activities and objectives personalized for each age group. As part of the promotion strategy, this program has a nationally distributed magazine (sold at newspaper shops) that features health care information related to these actions. In addition, television advertisements focus on healthy lifestyles, nutrition, obesity prevention, and promoting the magazine to the general public. Until now, this program has not been evaluated fully; however, a recent internal baseline survey was designed and implemented to assess the coverage of the main components and to evaluate intermediate program outcomes such as prevalence of anemia, frequency of physical activity, undernutrition, overweight, and obesity. This survey found an inadequate register of the nutritional status in the diverse population groups and of the health promotion activities. It is expected that one-year follow-up surveys will monitor selected outcomes of this integrated health program (Gutiérrez-Trujillo, 2005).

Ministry of Health Programs for Noncommunicable Chronic Diseases

The Ministry of Health of Mexico has several programs that consider prevention as a relevant component (Ministry of Health, 2006). These programs are not integrated health or nutrition programs but programs focused primarily on the most relevant public health problems, such as obesity, diabetes mellitus, high blood pressure, and cancer. Each of these diseases has a program that includes general management and preventive recommendations that must be followed by the government health service providers. However, most (if not all) of these programs, focus attention on promoting behavioral changes and early detection in adults, especially young adults over the age of 20 years. Obesity prevention during childhood and adolescence has been given much less consideration; rather, the predominant problems of concern for this group are related to food security (undernutrition and micronutrients deficiencies).

The following are some recently implemented actions for increasing the awareness and actions related to obesity prevention in children and youth in the public sector:

1. Implementation of regional or state-level programs; evaluation by the state (public) health sector needs to be conducted.
2. Creation of obesity clinics in public pediatric hospitals addressing the clinical care and management of obese children and research focuses on the consequences of obesity.
3. Development of an official memo outlining a future nationwide communication campaign for obesity prevention that in addition to addressing food production, media regulation, and food labeling, is intended to promote healthier lifestyles with special attention to children and adolescents.
4. Addition of obesity prevention among children and adolescents as one of the five priorities for research funding in the last request for proposals by CONACYT, the federal agency that provides oversight for research funding.

Moreover, recent efforts by the private sector have been implemented but must still be evaluated.

GOALS AND RECOMMENDATIONS

In accordance with the recommendations in the IOM report, *Preventing Childhood Obesity: Health in the Balance* (IOM, 2005), the final goals for obesity prevention among childhood and youth should be to stop the current trend in rising obesity incidence and prevalence and related chronic diseases and ultimately reduce the proportion of children and youth with an unhealthy weight. This ultimate goal necessarily should include increasing the proportion of children and adolescents meeting a healthful diet and appropriate amounts of regular physical activity and following a healthy growth trajectory. In the process of achieving these goals, it is important to define intermediate outcomes that will be needed to evaluate progress of a multi-faceted obesity prevention strategy. Based on the information described in previous sections, the authors propose a series of goals and recommendations for action for a multilevel and nationwide obesity prevention strategy among children and adolescents. An objective of the U.S.–Mexico binational meeting will be to broadly discuss this list of recommendations among key persons from each sector (e.g., academia, government, industry, schools, communities) to reach consensus on the next steps needed to initiate this multilevel strategy. A list of possible intermediate outcomes and goals for discussion during the binational meeting include:

• Increased quantity and quality of physical activity at schools in both planned physical education time and recreational time such as recess.
• Increased and improved facilities for recreational activities in communities, especially suburban areas.
• Increased advertising and marketing messages in preferably broadcast, cable, and satellite television, but also in other media such as radio, the Internet, and cell phones, aimed at children, youth, and their parents that promote healthy lifestyles, including healthful diets and regular physical activity.
• Decreased number of media advertising or marketing campaigns promoting high-calorie and low-nutrient food and beverage products targeted at children and adolescents that increase the risk of positive energy balance (such as refined sugars and saturated and *trans* fats).
• Decreased proportion of children and youth who have more than two hours of leisure screen time (including television and video watching) per day.
• Increased proportion of children and youth consuming more than five portions of fruits and vegetables per day.

As stated in the IOM recommendations, in order to achieve these types of intermediate outcomes, a multilevel strategy clearly is needed. However, in contrast to the U.S. context, Mexican society at large (e.g., government, industry, community leaders, schools, families) is far behind on some fundamental aspects needed to build support for this strategy. Three main issues that should be covered as priority steps in developing an effective obesity prevention strategy are:

• creating awareness among decision makers (including all branches of federal and state powers) as well as among the general public;
• regulating and enforcing laws;
• empowering communities so that they can achieve the necessary changes in different environments (e.g., school, community, industry) that, as described in previous sections, are contributing to a net positive energy balance among Mexicans in general, and specifically children and youth.

Priority recommendations for action specifically related to the Mexican context are listed below. The recommendations can be viewed as preliminary and will be modified through discussion with different stakeholders.

Government Level

• Underpin the idea of childhood obesity prevention as an urgent national priority, with strong participation and leadership of government at all levels in several actions including:

o Regulations and implementation of media and food, beverage, and restaurant industry policies;

o Support and funding of obesity prevention programs at federal and state levels with planned evaluations of their health impact;

o Support and funding of surveillance and monitoring efforts and wide dissemination of their findings not only at the national level, such as the National Nutrition Surveys, but also at the state and county levels;

o Planning of urban development with an appropriate access and promotion of facilities for recreational activities;

o Initiation of a widespread nationwide media campaign across print, electronic (e.g., radio, television), and wireless and Internet-based media (e.g., cell phones) to increase awareness of the obesity problem in the population;

o Expand the training of professionals to design, implement, and evaluate strategies for effectively responding to the obesity epidemic.

- Review current regulations for food labeling (NOM 051-SECOFI and NOM-086-SSA1-1994), evaluate the impact and consumers' understanding of food labeling, and make necessary modifications required to support obesity prevention goals.
- Review current government regulations and guidelines on the use of health claims on food products, especially nutrition-related health claims.
- Develop incentives or regulations for advertising and marketing to children and youth, especially for food and beverage products high in total calories and in particular for those with a high content of refined carbohydrates, added sugars, and fat.
- Seek mechanisms such as incentives or regulations to improve the enforcement of policies related to media and the food, beverage, and restaurant industries, including food labeling.
- Create an advisory committee that, together with the Federal Commission for the Protection from Sanitary Risk (COFEPRIS), will develop and evaluate policies for food labeling, marketing, media control, and dietary guidelines. This committee should include experts from different public and private institutions, as well as industry representatives and consumers. Priority steps should focus on the following areas:

o Modify food labeling, focusing on the need of acceptance and understanding for the majority of the population. Limited evidence suggests that most of the information contained on food labels is difficult for consumers to understand. Develop communication strategies that are clear and understandable by the general public.

o Reduce, at minimum, the content of health claims in media-based marketing, especially for those foods that promote "healthy" choices that do not meet basic nutritional guidelines.

o Conduct research on advertising and marketing targeted at Mexican children and youth focused on high-calorie, low-nutrient food and beverage products, and limit or eliminate practices that promote these types of products.

o In collaboration with industry, conduct research on the types and amount of fat that is used and needed in products.

o Set a limit on the recommended use of dietary fats and oils, particularly saturated fat and *trans* fats, by the food, beverage, and restaurant industry and fast food available through informal establishments.

o Regulate media marketing for food products with high content of refined carbohydrates and fat in regards to type of information, and advertising locations. For example, the possibility of setting strict limits in children's environments, such as schools, parks, and entertainment centers, should be researched and discussed.

- Evaluate the use of policy instruments such as international trade, subsidies, and taxes for encouraging or discouraging the production and consumption of certain foods to encourage the availability and access to healthful foods such as fruits and vegetables during all seasons and to reduce the consumption of less healthful foods and beverages.
- Promote the consumption of fruits and vegetables and other familiar healthful foods and beverages through diverse media.
- Promote a diverse media campaign supporting the consumption of water as a substitute for sweetened beverages (including carbonated soft drinks).

School Level

- Revise the school breakfast program to ensure healthful food and meal options.
- Regulate the foods and beverages offered to children and youth in and around the school environment.
- Promote the enforcement of minimally established time that children and youth participate in physical education in both private and public schools, as well as physical education programs that achieve the recommended amounts of moderate to vigorous physical activity.
- Encourage the organization of local and regional events to promote sports practice in schools.
- Define minimal spaces at schools to ensure regular physical activity during physical education time and during recess.
- Revise and improve school curricula to include obesity prevention and healthy lifestyle promotion.

Community Level

- Stimulate community organization and community members' empowerment to request and influence the modification of norms and environments aimed at achieving healthy lifestyles.
- Explore the spectrum of available organizations to identify the best strategies for increasing community empowerment and awareness, especially among parents, of the obesity epidemic. Potential community organizations include parents' societies, religious groups, and non-governmental organizations.

In conclusion, Mexico is on the course of an epidemiologic and nutritional transition toward more sedentary lifestyles and obesogenic environments. The present trajectory is moving toward an increasing burden of obesity in children and youth with serious predictable health and economic burdens to the entire population and Mexican society. These risks must be addressed immediately with multi-level interventions undertaken by a variety of stakeholders in government, schools, and communities targeting children and youth in many settings. The response to the growing obesity epidemic in Mexico will require many years and perhaps decades to implement and to evaluate the effectiveness of the results. The joint U.S.–Mexico workshop, for which this and the companion paper from the U.S. context served as background for discussion, should delineate the initial steps of the strategy required to tackle this urgent public health problem.

REFERENCES

Alsea. 2004. *Annual Report.* [Online.] Available: http://www.alsea.com.mx [accessed May 5, 2006].

Arredondo A, Zuñiga A. 2004. Economic consequences of epidemiologic changes in diabetes in middle-income countries: The Mexican case. *Diabetes Care* 27(1):104–109.

Arochi R, Tessmann KH, Galindo O. 2004. Advertising to children in Mexico. *Young Consumers* 6(4):82–85.

Bandini LG, Must A, Cyr H, Anderson SE, Spadano JL, Dietz WH. 2003. Longitudinal changes in the accuracy of reported energy intake in girls 10–15 years of age. *American Journal of Clinical Nutrition* 78(3):480–484.

Barker DJ. 1992. Fetal growth and adult disease. *British Journal of Obstetrics and Gynaecology* 99(4):275–276.

Barquera S, Rivera-Dommarco J, Safdie M, Flores-Aldana M, Campos-Nonato I, Campirano F. 2003. Energy and nutrient intake in pre-school and school-age Mexican children: National Nutrition Survey 1999. *Salud Pública de México* 45(4):540–550.

Barquera S, Hotz C , Rivera J, Tolentino L, Espinoza J, Campos I, Shamah T. In press. Food consumption, food expenditure, anthropometric status, and nutrition-related diseases in Mexico. In: Kennedy et al., eds. *Double-Burden of Malnutrition in Developing Countries.* Rome, Italy: Food and Agricultural Organization. Pp. 161–204.

Bray GA, Nielsen SJ, Popkin BM. 2004. Consumption of high-fructose corn syrup in beverages may play a role in the epidemic of obesity. *American Journal of Clinical Nutrition* 79:537–543.

Brewis A. 2003. Biocultural aspects of obesity in young Mexican school children. *American Journal of Human Biology* 15:446–460.

Caballero B. 2001. Early nutrition and risk of disease in the adult. *Public Health Nutrition* 4(6a):1335–1336.

Campirano F, Barquera S, Haas J, Téllez-Rojo M, Rivera-Dommarco J. 2003. Estimación del sub-reporte de energía en mujeres mexicanas obesas y no obesas. In: Barquera S, ed. *Aspectos de Alimentación y Nutrición en México*. Cuernavaca, México: Instituto Nacional de Salud Pública. Pp. 24–33.

Chagnon VC, Wilmore JH, Borecki IB. 2000. Association between the leptin receptor gene and adiposity in middle-aged Caucasian males from the heritage family study. *Journal of Clinical Endocrinology and Metabolism* 85:29–34.

Champagne CM, Baker NB, DeLany JP, Harsha DW, Bray GA. 1998. Assessment of energy intake underreporting by doubly labeled water and observations on reported nutrient intakes in children. *Journal of the American Dietetic Association* 98(4):426–433.

COFETEL (Comisión Federal de Telecomunicaciones). 2005. *Dirección General de Tarifas e Integración Estadística*. [Online]. Available: http://www.inegi.gob.mx [accessed November 11, 2005].

Cruz M, Torres M, Aguilar-Herrera B, Perez-Johnston R, Guzman-Juarez N, Aranda M, Kumate J. 2004. Type 2 diabetes mellitus in children—an increasing health problem in Mexico. *Journal of Pediatric Endocrinology and Metabolism* 17(2):183–190.

Du S, Mroz TA, Zhai F, Popkin BM. 2004. Rapid income growth adversely affects diet quality in China—particularly for the poor. *Social Science and Medicine* 59(7):1505–1515.

Fernald LC, Gutiérrez JP, Neufeld LM, Olaiz G, Bertozzi SM, Mietus-Snyder M, Gertler PJ. 2004. High prevalence of obesity among the poor in Mexico. *Journal of the American Medical Association* 291(21):2544-2545.

Fernandez JR, Shiver MD. 2004. Using genetic admixture to study the biology of obesity traits and to map genes in admixed populations. *Nutrition Review* 62(7):S69–S74.

Friedman AE, Dickler H. 2003. *International Advertising Clearance*. Amsterdam, Netherlands: Global Advertising Lawyers Alliance.

Friend B, Stapylton-Smith M. 1999. *Through the Eyes of Children*. Presentation at the ESOMAR Marketing in Latin America Conference. Santiago, Chile. April 1999.

Frongillo EA, de Onis M, Hanson KM. 1997. Socioeconomic and demographic factors are associated with worldwide patterns of stunting and wasting of children. *Journal of Nutrition* 127(12):2302–2309.

Gardner LI, Stern MP, Haffner SM, Gaskill SP, Hazuda HP, Relethford JH, Eifler CW. 1984. Prevalence of diabetes in Mexican Americans: Relationship to percent of gene pool derived from native American sources. *Diabetes* 33(1):86–92.

González-Castell D, Rivera-Dommarco J, González-Cossío T, Barquera-Cervera S. 2003. *Contribución de los alimentos industrializados en la ingestión de energía, macronutrimentos y fibra en niños mexicanos de 1 a 4 años*. M.S. Thesis. Cuernavaca, Morelos, México: Escuela de Salud Pública de México, Instituto Nacional de Salud Pública.

Gortmaker SL, Must A, Sobol AM, Peterson K, Colditz GA, Dietz WH. 1996. Television viewing as a cause of increasing obesity among children in the United States, 1986–1990. *Archives of Pediatrics and Adolescent Medicine* 150(4):356–362.

Gutiérrez-Trujillo G. 2005. Cobertura de los programas integrados de salud (PREVENIMSS): Promoción de la salud, nutrición, salud reproductiva, prevención, detección y control de enfermedades. In: Martínez-Salgado et al., eds. *Las Múltiples Facetas de la Investigación en Salud*. Instituto Mexicano del Seguro Social. Pp. 91–114.

Gutiérrez JP, Gertler P, Hernández Avila M, Bertozzi S. 2005. Impacto de Oportunidades en los comportamientos de riesgo de los adolescentes y en sus consecuencias inmediatas. Resultados de corto plazo en zonas urbanas y de mediano plazo en zonas rurales. In: Hernández Prado B, Hernández Avila M., eds. *Evaluación Externa de Impacto del Programa Oportunidades 2004*. Vol II. Cuernavaca, México: Instituto Nacional de Salud Pública Pp. 77–120.

Habicht JP, Martorell R, Yarbrough C, Malina RE, Klein RE. 1974. Height and weight standards for preschool children. How relevant are ethnic differences in growth potential? *Lancet* 1(7858):611–614.

Hales CN, Barker DJ. 2001. The thrifty genotype hypothesis. *British Medical Bulletin* 60: 5–20.

Hawkes C. 2002. Marketing activities of global soft drink and fast food companies in emerging markets: A review. In: *Globalization, Diets, and Non-Communicable Diseases*. Geneva, Switzerland: World Health Organization.

Hernández B, Gortmaker SL, Colditz GA, Peterson KE, Laird NM, Parra-Cabrera S. 1999. Association of obesity with physical activity, television programs and other forms of video viewing among children in Mexico City. *International Journal of Obesity* 23:845–854.

Hernández B, de Haene J, Barquera S, Monterrubio E, Rivera J, Shamah T, Sepúlveda J, Haas J, Campirano F. 2003. Factores asociados con la actividad física en mujeres mexicanas en edad reproductiva. *Rev Panam Salud Pública/Pan American Journal of Public Health* 14(4):235–245.

Horton ES. 1983. Introduction: An overview of the assessment and regulation of energy balance in humans. *American Journal of Clinical Nutrition* 38(6):972–977.

INEGI (Instituto Nacional de Estadística, Geografía e Informática). 2000. *Estados Unidos Mexicanos. XII Censo General de Población y Vivienda 2000. Base de Datos de la Muestra Censal, Cuestionario Ampliado, México*. [Online]. Available: http://www.inegi.gob.mx [accessed November 11, 2005].

INEGI. 2005a. *Encuesta Nacional sobre Disponibilidad y Uso de Tecnología de la Información y Comunicaciones en los Hogares*. [Online]. Available: http://www.inegi.gob.mx [accessed November 11, 2005].

INEGI. 2005b. *Estadísticas de Transportes*. [Online]. Available: http://www.inegi.gob.mx [accessed November 11, 2005].

IOM (Institute of Medicine). 2001. *Dietary Reference Intakes. Vitamin A, Vitamin K, Arsenic, Boron, Chromium, Copper, Iodine, Iron, Manganese, Molybdenum, Nickel, Silicon, Vanadium, and Zinc*. Washington, DC: National Academy Press.

IOM. 2005. *Preventing Childhood Obesity: Health in the Balance*. Washington, DC: The National Academies Press.

Kuczmarski RJ, Ogden CL, Grummer-Strawn LM, Flegal KM, Guo SS, Wei R, Mei Z, Curtin LR, Roche AF, Johnson CL. 2000. CDC growth charts. *Advanced Data* 314:1–27.

Lucas A, Fewtrell MS, Cole TJ. 1999. Fetal origins of adult disease—the hypothesis revisited. *British Medical Journal* 319:245–249.

McDonald's Corporation. 2006. *McDonald's 20 Años Conmigo*. [Online]. Available: http://www.mc20.com.mx [accessed May 5, 2006].

Mei Z, Grummer-Strawn L, Pietrobelli A, Goulding A, Goran M, Dietz W. 2002. Validity of body mass index compared with other body-composition screening indexes for the assessment of body fatness in children and adolescents. *American Journal of Clinical Nutrition* 75:978–985.

Ministry of Health. 2006. *Secretaria de Salud*. [Online]. Available: http://www.salud.gob.mx [accessed May 7, 2006].

Monterrubio-Flores EA. 2006. Curvas percentilares de talla edad de niños mexicanos de 2 a 9 años con características sociodemográficas asociadas a un buen crecimiento: Datos de la ENN II. M.S. Thesis. *Escuela de Salud Publica de México*. Instituto Nacional de Salud Pública, Cuernavaca, Morelos, México.

Neel JV. 1962. Diabetes mellitus: A "thrifty" genotype rendered detrimental by "progress"? *American Journal of Human Genetics* 14:353–362.

Neufeld L, García-Guerra A, Leroy F, Flores López ML, Fernández Gaxiola AC, Rivera-Dommarco JA. 2005. *Impacto del Programa Oportunidades en Nutrición y Alimentación en Zonas Urbanas de México*. [Online]. Available: http://evaloportunidades.insp.mx/441c7c1a3d30adf64e0e724174a9d527/impacto/2005/insp_2005_nutricion.pdf [accessed November 10, 2006].

Neufeld LM, Dominguez-Islas C, García-Guerra A, García-Feregrino R, Rivera-Dommarco J. 2006. Increase in body mass index over a two year period in women from urban Mexico. Experimental Biology Meeting, San Francisco, April 1–5. *Experimental Biology 2006 Meeting Program*. Abstract 638.7. P. 988.

Neufeld L, Sotres-Alvarez D, García-Feregrino R, García-Guerra A, Tolentino-Mayo L, Fernald L, Rivera-Donmarco J. 2005. Estudio comparativo sobre el estado nutricional y la adquisición de lenguaje entre niños de localidades urbanas con y sin Oportunidades. In: Hernández B, Hernández-Ávila M, eds. *Evaluación Externa de Impacto del Programa Oportunidades 2004, Tomo III*. Alimentación. México, D.F. Pp. 89–115.

Norma Oficial Mexicana. 2005. NOM-043-SSA2-2005, Servicios básicos de salud. Promoción y educación para la salud en materia alimentaria. Criterios para brindar orientación.

OECD (Organisation for Economic Co-operation and Development). 2005. OECD Health Data 2005. *How Does Mexico Compare?* [Online]. Available: http://www.oecd.org/dataoecd/16/2/34970198.pdf [accessed January 15, 2006].

Oksanen L, Ohman M, Heiman M. 1997. Markers for the gene ob and serum leptin levels in human morbid obesity. *Human Genetics* 99:559–564.

Olaiz G, Rojas R, Barquera S, Shamah T, Aguilar C, Cravioto P, Lopez P, Hernández M, Tapia R, Sepúlveda J. 2003. La Salud de los Adultos. In: Sepúlveda, J, Ed. *Encuesta Nacional de Salud 2000, Tomo II*. Cuernavaca, Morelos, México: Instituto Nacional de Salud Pública.

Patrick H, Nicklas TA. 2005. A review of family and social determinants of children's eating patterns and diet quality. *Journal of the American College of Nutrition* 24(2):83–92.

Popkin BM. 2001. The nutrition transition and obesity in the developing world. *Journal of Nutrition* 131:871S–873S.

Resano-Pérez E, Méndez-Ramírez I, Shamah-Levy T, Rivera JA, Sepúlveda J. 2003. Methods of the 1999 National Nutrition Survey. *Salud Pública de México* 45 (4S):s558–s564.

Rich-Edwards JW, Colditz GA, Stampfer MJ, Willett WC, Gillman MW, Hennekens CH, Speizer FE, Manson JE. 1999. Birthweight and the risk for type 2 diabetes mellitus in adult women. *Annals of Internal Medicine* 130(4):278–284.

Rivera JA, Shamah-Levy T, Villalpando-Hernández S, González de Cossio T, Hernández-Prado B, Sepúlveda J. 2001. *Encuesta Nacional de Nutrición 1999. Estado Nutricional en Niños y Mujeres en México*. Cuernavaca, Morelos, México: Instituto Nacional de Salud Pública.

Rivera JA, Barquera S, Campirano F, Campos I, Safdie M, Tovar V. 2002. Epidemiological and nutritional transition in Mexico: Rapid increase of non-communicable chronic diseases and obesity. *Public Health Nutrition* 5(1A):113–122.

Rivera JA, Sepúlveda-Amor J. 2003. Conclusions from the Mexican National Nutrition Survey 1999: Translating results into nutrition policy. *Salud Pública de México* 45 (S4):S565–S575.

Rivera JA, Barquera S, González-Cossio T, Olaiz G, Sepúlveda J. 2004a. Nutrition transition in Mexico and in other Latin American countries. *Nutrition Review* 62(7):S149–S157.

Rivera JA, Sotres-Alvarez D, Habicht JP, Shamah T, Villalpando S. 2004b. Impact of the Mexican program for education, health, and nutrition (Progresa) on rates of growth and anemia in infants and young children: A randomized effectiveness study. *Journal of the American Medical Association* 291(21):2563–2570.

Robinson TN. 2001. Television viewing and childhood obesity. *Pediatric Clinics of North America* 48(4):1017–1025.

Rodríguez-Moran M, Salazar-Vazquez B, Violante R, Guerrero-Romero F. 2004. Metabolic syndrome among children and adolescents aged 10–18 years. *Diabetes Care* 27(10):2516–2517.

Rosenbaum M, Leibel R. 1998. The physiology of body weight regulation. Relevance to the etiology of obesity in children. *Pediatrics* 101:525–539.

Secretaría de Comunicaciones y Transportes, *Dirección General de Sistemas de Radio y Televisión*. 2005. [Online]. Available: http://www.inegi.gob.mx [accessed November 11, 2005].

Secretaría de Educación Pública. 1994. Educación física. In: Fernández Editores SA de CV eds. *Educación Básica Primaria, Plan y Programas de Estudio*. México. D.F.: Pp. 149–162.

SEDESOL (Secretaría de Desarrollo Social). 2006. Oportunidades, reglas de operación 2006 Mexico DF, Secretaria de desarrollo social: Programa Oportunidades.

Seidell JC. 2000. Obesity, insulin resistance, and diabetes—A worldwide epidemic. *British Journal of Nutrition* 83:S5–S8.

Simmons R. 2005. Perinatal programming of obesity. *Experimental Gerontology* 40:863–866.

Snyder EE, Brandon W, Perusse L, Chagnon S, Weinagel J, Rankinen T, Bouchard C. 2004. The human obesity gene map: The 2003 update. *Obesity Research* 12(3):369–439.

Stein AD, Ravelli AC, Lumey LH. 1995. Famine, third-trimester pregnancy weight gain, and intrauterine growth: The Dutch Famine Birth Cohort Study. *Human Biology* 67(1): 135–150.

Stein AD, Conlisk A, Torin B, Schroeder DG, Grajeda R, Martorell R. 2002. Cardiovascular disease risk factors are related to adult adiposity but not birth weight in young Guatemalan adults. *Journal of Nutrition* 132(8):2208–2214.

Stern MP, Bartley M, Duggirala R, Bradshaw B. 2000. Birth weight and the Metabolic Syndrome: Thrifty phenotype or thrifty genotype? *Diabetes Metabolism Research and Reviews* 16:88–93.

Swallen KC, Reither EN, Haas SA, Meier AM. 2005. Overweight, obesity, and health-related quality of life among adolescents: The National Longitudinal Study of Adolescent Health. *Pediatrics* 115(2):340–347.

Trowbridge R, Mendoza F. 2007. Preventing obesity in Mexican–American children and youth. In: Institute of Medicine (IOM). *Joint U.S.–Mexico Workshop on Preventing Obesity in Children and Youth of Mexican Origin*. Washington, DC: The National Academies Press.

Uauy R, Albala C, Kain J. 2001. Obesity trends in Latin America: Transiting from under- to overweight. *Journal of Nutrition* 131:893S–899S.

Villa-Caballero L, Caballero-Solano V, Chavarria-Gamboa M, Linares-Lomeli P, Torres-Valencia E, Medina-Santillan R, Palinkas LA. 2005. *American Journal of Preventive Medicine* 30(3):197–203.

Villalpando S, García-Guerra A, Ramírez-Silvia CI, Mejía-Rodríguez F, Matute G, Shamah T, Rivera JA. 2003a. Iron, zinc and iodine status in Mexican children under 12 years and women 12–49 years of age: A probabilistic national survey. *Salud Pública de México* 45 (4S):S520–S529.

Villalpando S, Montalvo-Velarde I, Zambrano N, García-Guerra A, Ramírez-Silva CI, Shamah T, Rivera JA. 2003b. Vitamins A and C and folate status in Mexican children under 12 years and women 12–49 years: A probabilistic national survey. *Salud Pública de México* 45(4S):S508–S519.

Villalpando S, Shamah-Levy T, Ramírez-Silva CI, Mejía-Rodríguez F, Rivera JA. 2003c. Prevalence of anemia in children 1 to 12 years of age: Results from a nation-wide probabilistic survey in Mexico. *Salud Publica de Mexico* 45(4S):S490–S498.

Villalpando S, Carrión C, Barquera S. In press. The body mass index is associated with hyperglycemia and alterations of some components of the metabolic syndrome in Mexican adolescents aged 10–19 years. *Salud Pública de México.*

Villareal-Calderón A, Acuna H, Villareal-Calderon J. Garduno M, Henriquez-Roldan CF, Calderon-Garciduenas L, Valencia Salazar G. 2002. Assessment of physical education time and alter-school outdoor time in elementary and middle school students in south Mexico city: The dilemma between physical fitness and the adverse health effects of outdoor pollutant exposure. *Archives of Environmental Health* 57(5):451.

WHO (World Health Organization). 2004. *Global Strategy on Diet, Physical Activity, and Health.* Report No. WHA57.17. [Online]. Available: http://www.who.int/gb/ebwha/pdf_files/WHA57/A57_R17-en.pdf [accessed May 7, 2006].

WHO (World Health Organization). 2006a. *The WHO Child Growth Standards.* [Online]. Available: http://www.who.int/childgrowth/en [accessed May 5, 2006].

WHO. 2006b. *Preventing Chronic Diseases: A Vital Investment.* World Health Organization: Geneva, Switzerland. [Online]. Available: http://www.who.int/chp/chronic_disease_report/full_report.pdf [accessed May 5, 2006].

WARC (World Advertising Research Center). 2005. *The Americas Marketing Pocket Book 2005.* Oxfordshire, UK: WARC.

WCRF (World Cancer Research Fund). 1997. *Food, Nutrition, and the Prevention of Cancer: A Global Perspective.* Washingtron, DC: American Institute for Cancer Research.

Zahniser S, Young E, Wainio J. 2005. *Recent Agricultural Policy Reforms in North America.* Economic Research Service, U.S. Department of Agriculture WRS-05-03. [Online]. Available: http://www.ers.usda.gov/publications/WRS0503/wrs0503.pdf [accessed May 8, 2006].

C

Preventing Obesity in Mexican-American Children and Adolescents

Frederick Trowbridge, Trowbridge & Associates, Inc., Atlanta, Georgia
Fernando Mendoza, Stanford University School of Medicine Palo Alto, California

INTRODUCTION

Childhood obesity has become a worldwide concern because of its epidemic proportions and its growing link to type 2 diabetes and other chronic health conditions. Over the past two decades, there has been an increase in childhood and adolescent obesity to an unprecedented level. During the 1960s–1970s, the prevalence of obesity in children and adolescents in the United States was relatively stable at about 4–7 percent. However, during the 1980s the obesity prevalence doubled, with 11 percent of children and adolescents having body mass index (BMI) levels over the 95th percentile by the early 1990s (CDC, 2005b). In the latest National Health and Nutrition Examination Survey (NHANES) 2003–2004 (Ogden et al., 2006), childhood and adolescent obesity prevalence increased to 17 percent, which is triple the rate in NHANES I (1971–1974) and NHANES II (1976–1980) (Hedley et al., 2004). This dramatic increase in prevalence has driven childhood and adolescent obesity to a prominent position in the clinical and research arenas of child health. Moreover, as the links between obesity and its co-morbidities (e.g., type 2 diabetes, asthma, hypertension, sleep apnea, skeletal-muscular disorders, self-esteem and mental health disorders, and other chronic illnesses) have become more evident, the awareness of the long-term health effects of child and adolescent obesity has raised concerns at all levels of child health policy.

Addressing the problem of obesity in Mexican–American children and adolescents will require consideration of the unique historical and demographic characteristics of Mexican Americans. Since the 1500s Mexican Americans have lived in what is now the southwestern United States and have maintained a continuing interchange of culture with Mexico. Today, Mexicans continue to immigrate to locations across the United States, and to maintain their cultural ties. Currently, one in five children in the United States lives in an immigrant family; they are either first- or second-generation children of immigrant parents (NRC/IOM, 1998). The country of origin for the largest proportion of these children is Mexico. In 2000, 39 percent of children in families new to the United States were Mexican—no other country contributes more than 4 percent (Hernandez, 2004).

The substantial and ongoing interchange of people and culture between the United States and Mexico makes it clear that addressing childhood obesity in the Mexican–American community requires an approach that recognizes the common social, cultural, economic, and possibly genetic factors that contribute to childhood obesity in both Mexican–American and Mexican children and adolescents. At the same time, the influence of the substantially different social, cultural, and economic environment in which Mexican–Americans living in the United States find themselves, must also be taken into account. This paper reviews the prevalence and trends in obesity in Mexican–American children and youth and considers the multiple factors that may contribute to this growing health problem. The paper then provides an overview of current intervention strategies and programs and proposes actions that may offer the greatest potential for success in preventing and controlling the obesity epidemic.

EXTENT AND CONSEQUENCES OF OBESITY IN MEXICAN–AMERICAN CHILDREN AND YOUTH

Data from national surveys clearly demonstrate a high and increasing prevalence of childhood obesity in the United States (Ogden et al., 2002, 2006; Hedley et al., 2004). Obesity is particularly prevalent among Mexican–American children and youth. Moreover, Mexican–American children have a high prevalence of abdominal obesity, which may put them at elevated risk for type 2 diabetes and cardiovascular disease (CVD). High rates of obesity also may indicate that Mexican–American children and adolescents are more exposed to the negative impacts of obesity on their social and emotional health. Finally, since many Mexican–American children and youth depend on publicly funded health care programs such as Medicaid, the high prevalence of obesity will place increasing demands on health care providers serving Hispanic populations and thus will have significant implications for the funding needs of these programs.

Measurement of Obesity in Children and Youth

Body Mass Index (BMI)

BMI is recommended widely as an appropriate measure of obesity in children older than 2 years of age (Daniels et al., 1997; Pietrobelli et al., 1998). This indicator is calculated easily from simple measurements of height and weight and is associated closely with indicators of cardiovascular disease (CVD) risk (Katzmarzyk et al., 2004). In addition, analysis of BMI data is facilitated by the availability of gender-specific reference data developed by the CDC for determining BMI-for-age percentiles (Kuczmarski et al., 2002). Reference curves based on an international data set derived from large, nationally representative surveys of child growth from six countries also are available (Cole et al., 2000). These reference curves are designed to merge smoothly with the BMI values for adults defining *overweight* as having a BMI between 25 to 29.9 kg/m^2 and *obese* as having a BMI equal to or greater than 30 kg/m^2. For consistency between the IOM report and this paper, obesity in children and youth is defined as having a BMI equal to or greater than age- and gender-specific 95th percentile of the BMI charts developed by the Centers for Disease Control and Prevention (CDC) in 2000. Being at-risk for obesity is defined as having a BMI between the age- and gender-specific 85th and 95th percentiles of the CDC BMI charts (IOM, 2005).

However, BMI also has recognized limitations as an obesity indicator. The relationship of BMI to body fat in children varies in relation to age, maturational stage, gender, race, and fat distribution, so that a given BMI will not reflect an equivalent level of body fat for all individuals (Daniels et al., 1997). Despite these limitations, BMI remains a useful and practical indicator for clinical assessment and for characterizing obesity prevalence in population-based studies.

Waist Circumference

Waist circumference is a more specific indicator of abdominal fat, and it appears to perform at least as well as BMI in identifying children with a clustering of CVD risk factors (Katzmarzyk et al., 2004). Among the 4–17-year-old children and youth who were sampled in the NHANES III (1988–1994), waist-to-height ratio actually performed better than BMI in identifying those with elevated CVD risk factors (Kahn et al., 2005). A 10-year cohort study beginning when children were 9 and 10 years old found that waist circumference and triglyceride level were significant predictors of the metabolic syndrome[1] at ages 18 to 19 years. In this study, BMI was not a

---

[1]The metabolic syndrome is diagnosed when an individual has at least three of five meta-

significant predictor once waist circumference was included in the multivariate model (Morrison et al., 2005). The importance of abdominal obesity as a risk factor for CVD in adults was highlighted in a recent study that found that having an elevated waist-to-hip ratio was associated more strongly with myocardial infarction than having an elevated BMI (Yusuf et al., 2005). The population-attributable risk of myocardial infarction for the top two quintiles of waist-to-hip ratio was 24.3 percent versus only 7.7 percent for the top two quintiles of BMI.

Descriptive data showing percentile distributions of waist circumference have been developed for 2–8-year-old African–American, European–American, and Mexican–American children based on data from NHANES III (Fernandez et al., 2004). In the same NHANES III data set, the waist circumference-to-height ratio did not vary significantly in relation to sex or age group, making it feasible to use a single set of cutoffs for classifying children of both sexes and all ages from 4 to 17 years (Kahn et al., 2005). The strong association of increased waist circumference with CVD risk factors and the availability of reference data support the use of waist circumference indicators, in addition to BMI, as valid and practical tools for assessing obesity and associated CVD risk in children and adolescents. However, additional research is needed to confirm the risks associated with abdominal obesity in different age, gender, and ethnic groups (especially Mexican and Mexican–American children and youth) and the usefulness of waist circumference as an indicator, alone or in combination with BMI, in identifying abdominal obesity in these different groups of children and adolescents.

Obesity Prevalence and Trends

Prevalence

Since the late 1970s, there has been a dramatic increase in the prevalence of obesity among children and youth across all racial and ethnic groups in the United States. Data from national surveys indicate that the prevalence of obesity has more than doubled for children ages 2–5 years and adolescents ages 12–19 years, and obesity rates have more than tripled for children ages 6–11 years (Ogden et al., 2002). Prevalence estimates based on the National Longitudinal Survey of Youth data from 1986–1998 in children ages 4–12 years provide a similar picture of the increasing prevalence of obesity (Strauss and Pollack, 2001).

---

bolic abnormalities: glucose intolerance, abdominal obesity, elevated triglyceride levels, low high-density lipoprotein levels, and high blood pressure.

An elevated prevalence of obesity is particularly evident for Mexican–American boys. In NHANES 2003–2004 (Ogden et al., 2006), Mexican–American boys ages 2–5 and 6–11 years had a higher prevalence of obesity than boys of any other race or ethnic group, while obesity prevalence for male adolescents was similar to other ethnic groups. (Figure C-1). In the 2003–2004 NHANES, Mexican–American girls ages 2–5 and 6–11 years had a prevalence of obesity that was less than that of African–American girls but greater than that of non-Hispanic White girls, while obesity prevalence for female Mexican–American adolescents was similar to non-Hispanic Whites (Figure C-2). Figure C-3 displays more data on obesity prevalence detailed by age group, gender, and ethnicity (Ogden et al., 2006). Additional research is needed to assess the underlying attitudes and diet and physical activity practices that may trigger these age, gender, and ethnic group differences.

It is of interest to compare the prevalence of obesity in Mexican–American children and adolescents with their counterparts in Mexico. Data from the Mexican National Nutrition Survey (1999) (Rivera et al., 2001) and the Mexican National Health Survey (2000) (Olaiz et al., 2003) were analyzed using the same CDC reference criteria to define obesity (López Ridaura et al., 2006; del Rio-Navarro et al., 2004; Kuczmarski et al., 2002). Overall, results indicated that, except for the preschool age group, Mexican children had a lower prevalence of obesity than ethnically similar children in the United States surveyed in 1999–2000 (Ogden et al., 2006). Obesity prevalence in 2–5-year-old Mexican children was similar to their

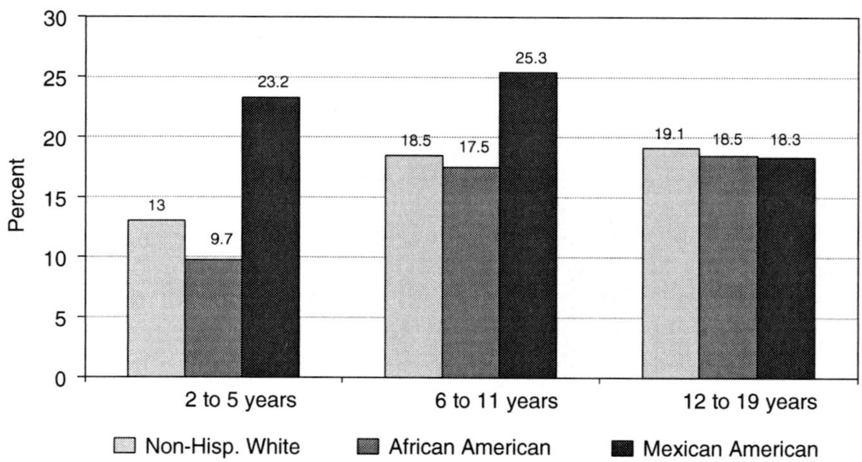

FIGURE C-1 Obesity prevalence in boys, NHANES 2003–2004.
SOURCE: Ogden et al. (2006).

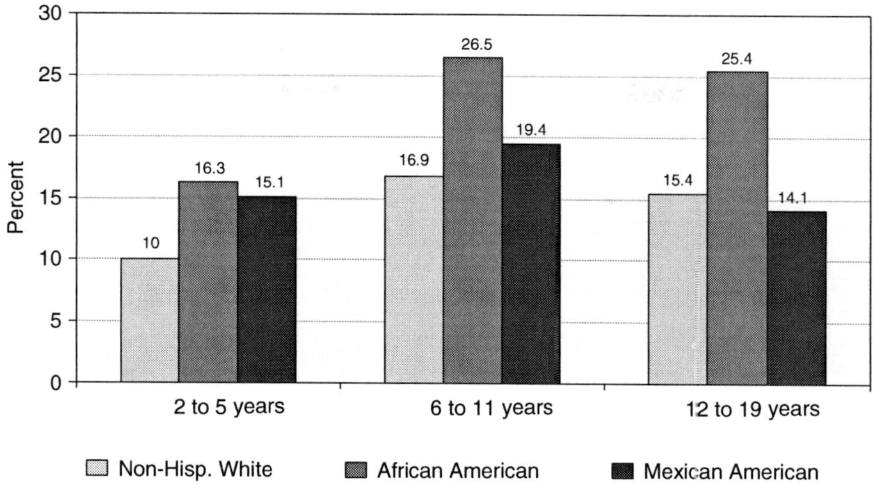

FIGURE C-2 Obesity prevalence in girls, NHANES 2003–2004.
SOURCE: Ogden et al. (2006).

Mexican–American counterparts. However, older Mexican children and adolescents had an obesity prevalence that was only half or one-third of the prevalence seen in Mexican–American children and adolescents (Table C-1 and Figure C-4).

These results in children and adolescents from ethnically similar backgrounds suggest that environmental factors in the United States exert a significant influence on the growth and weight status of Mexican–American children and youth.

Abdominal Obesity Prevalence

Abdominal obesity appears to be a particular concern for Mexican adults, children, and youth. Data from the Mexican National Health Survey conducted in 2000 indicate a high prevalence of abdominal obesity in Mexican adults based on waist circumference measurements, with a reported prevalence of 46.3 percent in men (waist circumference ≥ 94 cm) and 81.4 percent in women (waist circumference ≥ 80 cm) (Sanchez-Castillo et al., 2005). Abdominal obesity was elevated even in women of normal weight, with co-morbidities relating better to waist circumference than to BMI. Moreover, the high prevalence of abdominal obesity in Mexican men and women was associated with a prevalence of diabetes and hypertension similar to or exceeding levels observed in the non-Hispanic White population in NHANES III (1988–1994).

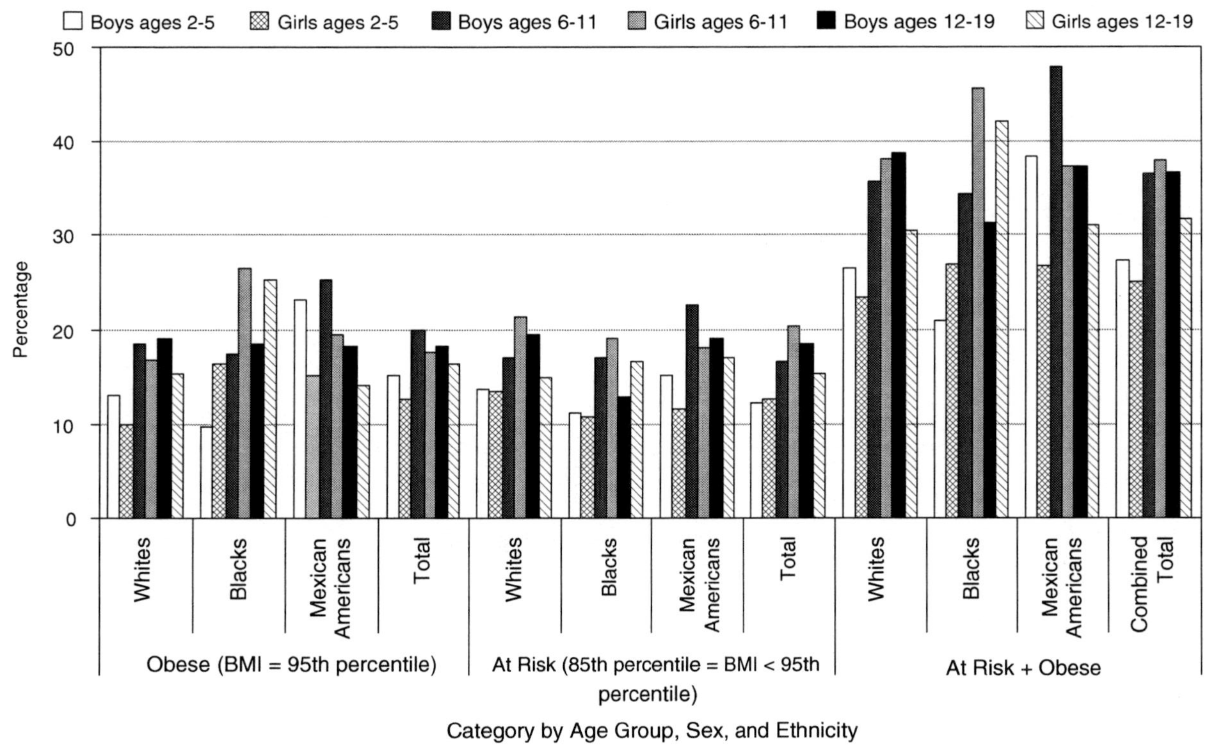

FIGURE C-3 Percentage of U.S. children and adolescents who are obese or at risk for obesity, by age, gender, and ethnicity, 2003–2004.
SOURCE: Ogden et al. (2006).

TABLE C-1 Prevalence of Obesity in Non-Hispanic White, Mexican–American, and Mexican Children: 1999–2000

Age/ Gender Group	NHANES 1999–2000 Non-Hispanic White	NHANES 1999–2000[a] Mexican American	Mexican National Nutrition Survey[b] 1999	Mexican National Health Survey[c] 2000
Boys				
2–5	6.9	13.1	11.1	
6–11	11.9	26.7	9.1	
12–17	11.8	27.2		10.6
Girls				
2–5	10.5	8.7	9.7	
6–11	11.6	19.8	8.5	
12–17	11.0	19.3		9.3

NOTE: Obesity is defined as greater than 95th percentile of BMI (Kuczmarski et al., 2002).
[a]Ogden et al. (2002).
[b]Rivera et al. (2002).
[c]del Rio-Navarro et al. (2004). Data represent average prevalence values for children 12 to 17 years.

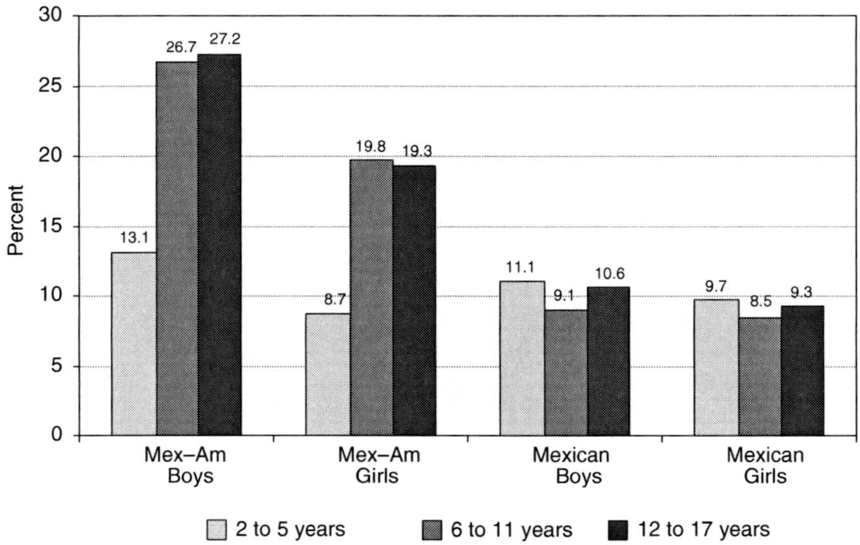

FIGURE C-4 Prevalence of obesity in Mexican–American and Mexican children, 1999–2000.
SOURCE: Rivera et al. (2002) and del Rio-Navarro et al. (2004).

These observations of increased abdominal obesity in Mexican adults parallel the finding of increased abdominal girth in Mexican–American children and youth. In the NHANES III survey, 13.9 percent of Mexican–American children were classified as having a waist circumference-to-height ratio category that exceeded their BMI category, whereas only 7 percent of non-Hispanic Blacks and 9.48 percent of the overall sample were so classified (Kahn et al., 2005). A separate analysis of NHANES III data found that the smoothed 90th percentile of waist circumference for Mexican–American boys was consistently higher than that observed for either African–American boys or European–American boys. The 90th percentile for Mexican–American girls also was consistently higher than that of European–American girls at all ages and greater than that of African–American girls up to 9 years of age. Analysis of waist circumference data from the 1999–2000 NHANES survey also found a consistent pattern of higher mean waist circumference values for Mexican–American children (Ford et al., 2004) (Figure C-5).

These findings of increased waist circumference suggest that Mexican–American children and youth, and particularly Mexican–American boys at all ages, may be at an increased risk of co-morbidities associated with abdominal obesity, including type 2 diabetes.

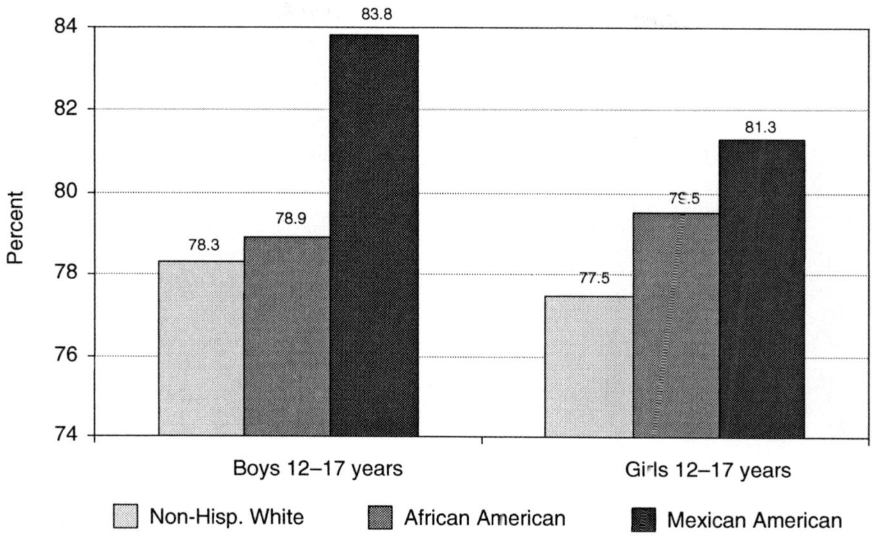

FIGURE C-5 Waist circumference (cm) of boys and girls 12–17 years old, by ethnic group.
SOURCE: NHANES 1999–2000; Ford et al. (2004).

Historical and Current Obesity Trends

Obesity among Mexican–American children is not a new finding. A review of growth studies on Mexican–American children and youth during 1920–1980 (based primarily on immigrant and low-income Mexican Americans) showed a high prevalence of short stature and low weight that was indicative of undernutrition (Malina et al., 1986). However, by the 1970s and early 1980s, regional studies in this review indicated a higher-than-expected level of obesity among Mexican–American children and youth. This increased level of obesity was associated with a shorter stature as compared with non-Hispanic Whites, resulting in a short, plump physique.

Data from NHANES I (1971–1974) demonstrated that differences in BMI between Mexican–American and non-Hispanic children and youth were related significantly to socioeconomic status (SES) (Mendoza and Castillo, 1986). Mexican–American children who had a lower SES had BMIs higher than their non-Hispanic counterparts, but this finding disappeared as SES increased. A combined analysis of NHANES I (1971–1974) and NHANES II (1976–1978) also found that stature was associated directly with SES and that poor children and youth were shorter (Martorell et al., 1988b). Overall, Mexican–American children and youth in this study were shown to have a short, plump physique, and the data suggested they also had increased upper body fat (Martorell et al., 1988a). Height comparisons between Mexican–American children and non-Hispanic White children showed differences related to SES, although a similar association was not seen for Mexican–American adolescents. These observations suggest that short stature in lower SES Mexican–American children was likely to be related to less adequate nutrition early in life or even during the prenatal period. Since an SES effect was not seen in adolescents it may be that other factors, possibly genetic, are more influential after puberty.

Data analysis from the Hispanic Health and Nutrition Examination Survey (HHANES) (1982–1984) indicated that Mexican–American children showed a higher-than-expected proportion of children above the 90th percentile for BMI between ages 6–11 years—with several year-groups showing twice the expected level—although adolescents showed more variability in the prevalence of obesity (Martorell et al., 1989). Further analyses of the HHANES showed that obesity was associated with increased centralized upper body adiposity and was not a result of having a different body proportion as compared with non-Hispanic Whites (Kaplowitz et al., 1989; Martorell et al., 1988a). In summary, data from HHANES confirmed findings from early studies, indicating that Mexican–American children had increased levels of obesity.

The upward trend in obesity prevalence in Mexican–American children has continued in recent years. Between NHANES III (1988–1994) and NHANES (2003–2004), the prevalence of obesity in adolescent Mexican–American boys ages 12–19 years increased by 4.2 percent (Figure C-6). Among girls, the largest increases were noted in non-Hispanic White and African–American adolescents, although obesity also increased in Mexican–American girls (Figure C-7) (NCHS, 2004; Ogden et al., 2006). It is interesting to note that reported obesity prevalence in male Mexican–American adolescents 12–19 years old decreased from 27.2 percent in 1999–2000 to 18.3 percent in 2003–2004, and in female adolescents from 19.3 percent in 1999–2000 to 14.1 percent in 2003–2004 (Ogden et al., 2006). The authors note that subgroup estimates by sex, age, and race/ethnicity are less precise than overall estimates due to smaller sample sizes, so that these prevalence estimates must be interpreted with caution.

It is interesting to note that as obesity prevalence has increased over the last several decades, the linear growth of Mexican–American children and adolescents has shown relatively little change. Linear growth improved from the 1960s to 1980s when HHANES was conducted, suggesting that Mexican–American children and youth had not previously been achieving their full height potential (Martorell et al., 1989). Analysis of more recent data indicates that although weight-for-age and BMI percentiles of Mexican–American children increased between HHANES (1982–

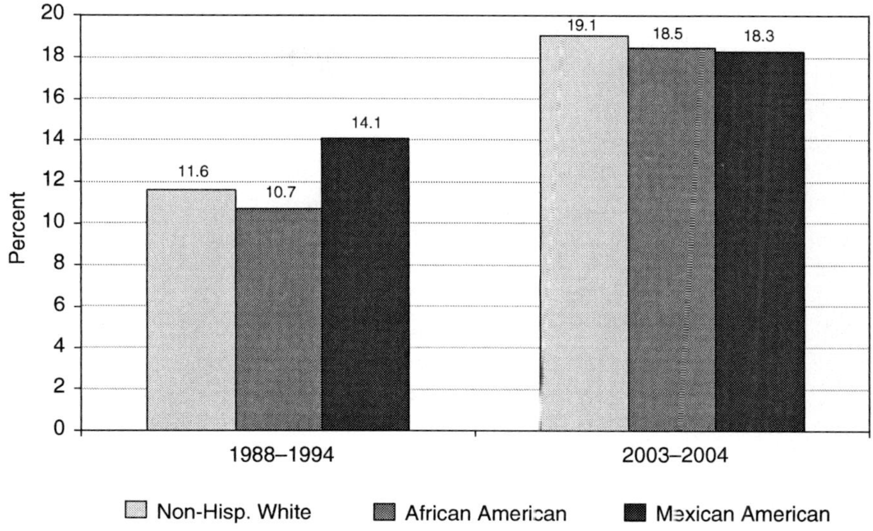

FIGURE C-6 Obesity trends in males 12–19 years old. NHANES 1988–1994 versus 2003–2004.
SOURCE: Table 70, Health, U.S. (2004); Ogden et al. (2006).

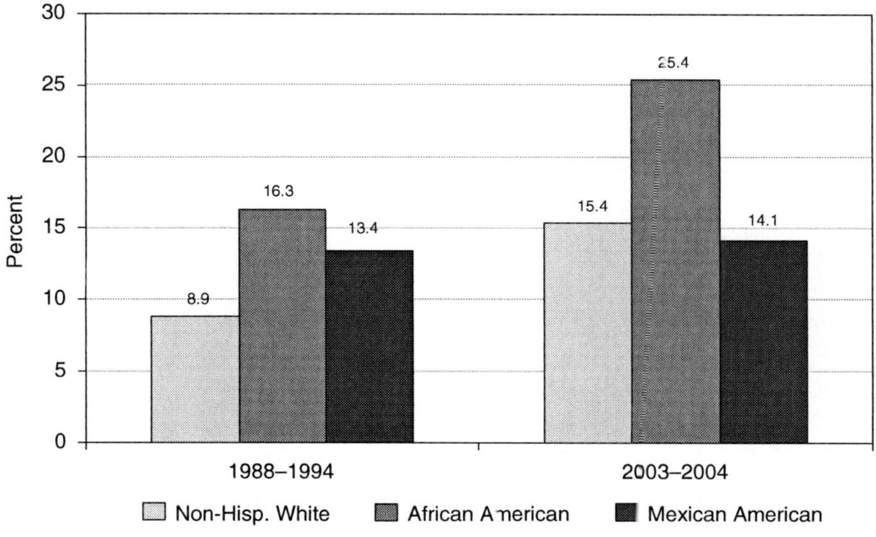

FIGURE C-7 Obesity trends in females 12–19 years old. NHANES 1988–1994 versus 2003–2004.
SOURCE: Table 70, Health, U.S. (2004); Ogden et al. (2006).

1984) and NHANES III (1988–1994), stature-for-age percentiles were largely unchanged (Ryan et al., 1999). Moreover, median height-for-age values for Mexican–American children in NHANES III closely paralleled the median of the CDC reference population and thus indicated that Mexican–American children were achieving linear growth similar to the general U.S. population up to early adolescence.

At approximately 13 to 14 years of age, however, the median stature of Mexican–American girls and boy falls to about the 25th percentile of the CDC reference. The reasons for the falloff in linear growth in adolescents are not well defined but might be related to genetic influences such as an earlier onset of puberty. In any case, the pattern of increased weight-for-age in the interval from HHANES to NHANES III, coupled with little change in stature-for-age, has resulted in a higher ratio of weight to height and is reflected in the increased prevalence of elevated BMI values in Mexican–American children and youth. Further research is needed to better understand the underlying causes of this pattern of linear and weight growth as well as the relationship it may have to the development of obesity. It also would be of interest to compare the pattern of weight and stature growth in Mexican–American children and adolescents with the pattern observed in their counterparts in Mexico.

Data from the National Longitudinal Survey of Youth also demonstrate the upward trend in childhood obesity and indicate a more rapid increase among Hispanic and African–American youth when compared to their European–American counterparts (Strauss and Pollack, 2001). Between 1986 and 1998, the annual rate of increase in obesity prevalence in children ages 4–12 years has been estimated at 4.3 percent and 5.8 percent for Hispanic and African–American youth, respectively, when compared to 3.2 percent for European–American youth. Obesity increased more rapidly among children in southern states (6.2 percent per year) when compared with children in northeastern, central, and western states (3.6 percent, 1.8 percent, and 2.2 percent, respectively) (Strauss and Pollack, 2001). This regional difference in prevalence may be related partly to the high prevalence of Hispanics residing in the southern United States.

Trends in waist circumference in children and adolescents also have been observed. In the interval between NHANES III (1988–1994) and NHANES (1999–2000), waist circumference increased significantly among 12–17-year-old adolescents (Ford et al., 2004). The largest increase in this age group was observed among Mexican–American boys, whose mean waist circumference measurements increased by 5.8 cm (from 78 cm to 83.8 cm)—an increase that was larger than that seen in African–American (5.2 cm) or White non-Hispanic boys (0.5 cm). The mean waist circumference of Mexican–American adolescent girls increased by 5 cm (from 76.3 cm to 81.3 cm)—an increase that was greater than that observed for African–American girls (2.9 cm) or European–American girls (3 cm) of the same age group. These findings indicate a significant increase in abdominal obesity among Mexican–American adolescents.

Overall, these data indicate that childhood obesity, and perhaps abdominal obesity in particular, represents a long-term and increasing problem among Mexican–American children and adolescents.

Health and Economic Impacts of Obesity

Impact on Physical Health

The relationship between obesity and chronic disease risk in adults has been observed and documented widely. Obesity increases the risk of many conditions including hypertension, CVD, stroke, type 2 diabetes, and certain types of cancer. Since obese children and youth are more likely to be overweight or obese as adults, there is a direct link between childhood obesity and long-term chronic disease risk. Concerns about childhood-onset obesity are supported by documented associations between childhood obesity and increased CVD risk and mortality in adulthood (Srinivasan et al., 2002; Li et al., 2004). Lifetime risk of developing type 2 diabetes for children born in the United States in 2000 has been estimated at 30 percent for boys and 40 percent for girls, with a higher level of risk for ethnic minorities (Narayan, 2003). Although childhood-onset obesity accounts for only 25 percent of adult obesity cases, obesity that is present before a child is 8 years of age and persists into adulthood is associated with severe obesity—defined as a BMI greater than 40 kg/m^2—in adulthood as compared with a BMI of 35 for adult-onset obesity (Freedman et al., 2001). Between 1990 and 2000, severe obesity (which is associated with more serious health complications) more than doubled, increasing from 0.78 percent to 2.2 percent in U.S. adults (Freedman et al., 2002).

Longitudinal data in 5–17-year-old European–American and African–American children indicate that obese children had a significantly increased risk for elevated low-density lipoprotein cholesterol, systolic and diastolic blood pressure, and fasting insulin. Fifty percent of the children with two or more of these risk factors were identified by using obesity (defined as a BMI equal to or greater than the 95th percentile) as a screening tool (Freedman et al., 1999). More recent studies in 126 obese Hispanic children ages 8–13 years found that 90 percent of these children had at least one feature of the metabolic syndrome and 30 percent had three or more risk factors and were diagnosed with the metabolic syndrome (Cruz et al., 2004). Furthermore, a recent analysis of NHANES (1999–2000) found that 12–19-year-old Mexican–American adolescents had a higher prevalence (13 percent) of impaired fasting glucose than either non-Hispanic Black (4.2 percent) or non-Hispanic White adolescents (7 percent) (Williams et al., 2005).

As noted previously, increased waist circumference or waist-to-height ratio have been shown to be as effective, or even more effective than BMI, in identifying children with multiple CVD risk factors (Katzmarzyk et al., 2004; Kahn et al., 2005). For this reason, the increasing abdominal obesity observed in Mexican–American youth indicates that they may be at particular risk for CVD in adulthood.

The association of obesity with the risk of developing type 2 diabetes in childhood and adolescence is a particularly serious concern. Children and adolescents who develop type 2 diabetes may experience the micro- and macrovascular complications of this disease at younger ages than individuals who develop diabetes in adulthood (Hannon et al., 2005). An increasing incidence of type 2 diabetes was documented in a longitudinal study from 1982–1994 that showed a 10-fold increase—from 0.7 cases per 100,000 per year in 1982 to 7.2 cases per 100,000 per year in 1994—in incidence among 10–19-year-old adolescents (Pinhas-Hamiel et al., 1996).

An analysis of data from NHANES III (1988–1994) and NHANES (1999–2002) showed a higher prevalence of diabetes and impaired glucose tolerance (a pre-diabetic condition) among Mexican–American adults compared with non-Hispanic Whites, which is consistent with data showing that Mexican–American adults are 1.7 times more likely to have diabetes than non-Hispanic White adults (CDC, 2003, 2005a). Similarly, higher rates of type 2 diabetes are being observed in Mexican–American children and adolescents. As an example, a survey of six high schools in Ventura County, California, identified 28 diabetic adolescents—75 percent more than expected (Neufeld et al., 1998). Correlations were found between the Hispanic enrollment in each school and the number of diabetic adolescents as well as between the obesity rates and adolescents with type 2 diabetes and impaired glucose tolerance.

Sleep apnea is another morbidity related to obesity. It has been suggested that Mexican Americans may have a higher prevalence of sleep apnea than other Hispanic subgroups (Strohl and Redline, 1996). Unfortunately, the available data for the prevalence of obstructive sleep apnea among Mexican–American children and adolescents are very limited (R. Pelayo, Stanford University Sleep Center, personal communication, 2005), even though clinical experience in obesity centers suggests that this is a prominent and growing problem (L. Hammer, Stanford University Medical Center, personal communication, 2005).

Asthma is another morbidity associated with childhood obesity. This condition has been reported to occur at a similar rate among Mexican–American children and adolescents surveyed in HHANES and NHANES III when compared with non-Hispanic Whites (NCR/IOM, 1998, 1999). An analysis by generational status of Mexican–American children and adolescents recorded a lower maternal-reported prevalence of asthma among first-

and second-generation children when compared with third and later generations (NRC/IOM, 1998). Although these data are self-reported and rely on having access to physicians, the trend of increasing asthma with each generation mirrors the pattern for childhood and adolescent obesity. An evaluation of the prevalence of asthma among Mexican–American children and youth in NHANES III showed an odds ratio of 2.1 (1.4, 2.9) for children with a BMI greater than the 85th percentile (Agredano et al., 2004).

Other physical conditions associated with obesity are abnormal serum lipids, hyperinsulinemia or glucose intolerance, and hypertension. These conditions form the basis for Syndrome X (also called the metabolic syndrome). A sample of 52 non-Hispanic White mother–child pairs were compared with 92 Mexican–American mother–child pairs to assess the risk for abnormal lipid profiles, hyperinsulinemia, hypertension, and obesity (Reaven et al., 1998). The findings of this study showed higher levels of obesity and hyperinsulinemia in Mexican–American children and adults compared with non-Hispanic White children and adults and therefore indicated that the Mexican Americans had an increased risk for CVD. Subsequent recommendations for avoiding increased rates of Syndrome X in Mexican American populations included early dietary intervention and exercise modification (Reaven et al., 1998).

Impact on Social and Emotional Health

In addition to the effects of obesity on physical health status and long-term chronic disease risk, obesity in childhood and adolescence can affect social and emotional well-being. As early as 5 years of age, higher weight status in girls was found to be associated with decreased body self-esteem and a perception of decreased cognitive abilities (Davidson and Birch, 2001). The same study found that independent of the girls' actual weight status a higher level of parental concern about child obesity was associated with a lower perception of physical and cognitive abilities by the daughters.

Another study among kindergartners and first-graders found that obesity was associated with lower academic performance in unadjusted data; however, after social and economic variables (e.g., race and ethnicity as well as mothers' education levels) were considered, the association was no longer significant (Datar and Magnabosco, 2004). These findings suggest that obesity is a marker but not a causal factor in children's academic performance. However, this study points out that obesity is observed more easily by other students compared with SES characteristics, and its significant association (unadjusted) with lower academic performance can contribute to the stigma of obesity, even in the early years of elementary school. Mexican–American children may experience a double burden of stigmatization because of the combined effects of stigmas associated with both obesity and ethnic origin.

Obese children are often subject to teasing from their normal-weight peers. The degree of teasing has been associated with higher weight concerns, more loneliness, poorer self-perception of physical appearance, higher preference for sedentary and isolated activities, and lower preference for physical or social activities (Hayden-Wade et al., 2005). Obesity also can affect self-perceived quality of life. A study of 106 children and adolescents ages 5–18 years (60 percent of the youth were Mexican) who were referred to a children's hospital for evaluation of obesity found that the self-reported quality of life score of the obese children and youth was significantly lower than that of their normal-weight peers and was similar to the score reported by children diagnosed with cancer (Schwimmer et al., 2003). Another study of body image and adolescent mental health found that Hispanic girls were more depressed and had lower self-esteem than other racial and ethnic groups even after controlling for body image. This study concluded that Hispanic adolescents may be at increased risk for mental health problems (Siegel et al., 1999).

Mexican–American children and adolescents have had a long battle with obesity and continue to lead the nation with regard to the proportion of their population who are either obese or at high risk for becoming obese. In addition, they are exhibiting the co-morbidities associated with obesity. Mexican–American adults are demonstrating the poor health outcomes associated with obesity, including increased levels of diabetes and CVD. It is important to remember that today's adults were children and adolescents in the 1970s and 1980s when Mexican Americans were first recognized to be at a greater risk for obesity. Consequently, if Mexican–American adults currently have some of the highest rates of diabetes in the country, what will this population look like when the current group of children become adults?

Impact on Health Care Costs

Studies of health care expenditures in the United States have documented the high cost and sharp upward trend in expenditures attributable to obesity. Econometric models indicate that the annual cost of obesity-related health care is approximately $75 billion (expressed in 2003 dollars) and that approximately half of these expenditures are financed by public funds through Medicare and Medicaid programs (Finkelstein et al., 2004). Overall, per capita health care costs have been rising rapidly, from an estimated $2,188 per capita in 1987 to $3,298 per capita in 2001 (expressed in 2001 dollars). Approximately 27 percent of this increase, or $301 per capita, can be attributed to obesity-related health care costs (Thorpe et al., 2004).

Hospital discharge data indicate that the economic burden of obesity-related illness is also increasing among children and youth in the United States. From 1979 to 1999 discharges with a diagnosis of diabetes nearly doubled, obesity and gallbladder diseases tripled, and sleep apnea discharges increased fivefold (Wang and Dietz, 2002). The same study also documented a greater than threefold increase in obesity-associated hospital costs, from $35 million during 1979–1981 to $127 million during 1997–1999.

These studies did not identify specifically health care costs associated with increasing obesity in Mexican-American children and youth. However, since many Mexican–American families depend on publicly funded programs (such as Medicaid) for health care, and since many may be underinsured or uninsured, the high prevalence and rapid increase in obesity among Mexican Americans inevitably will place increasing demands on these health care providers and have important implications for the funding needs of these programs (Flores et al., 1998; Burgos et al., 2005).

To date no study has calculated the economic impact of obesity in Mexican–American children and youth. However, an analysis of the economic impact of obesity has been conducted for the state of California, where approximately 35 percent of the population is Mexican American, 50 percent of the infants born are Hispanic and primarily Mexican American, and a large immigrant (mainly Mexican) population exists. This analysis assessed the economic cost attributable to physical inactivity, being overweight, and obesity with respect to medical costs, workers compensation, and loss productivity. The results showed a $21.7 billion loss—$10.2 billion in medical care, $338 million in workers compensation, and $11.2 billion in loss productivity. The following annual costs were determined: physical inactivity, $13.3 billion; obesity, $6.4 billon; and being overweight, $2 billion. An increase to $28 billion by 2005 subsequently was forecast unless aggressive actions were taken (Chenoweth, 2005).

These data from California provide insight into the enormous economic costs associated with obesity. When these costs are projected to the national level in the United States and Mexico, the overall impact on health care costs is staggering. Moreover, the outlook is that these costs will continue to increase unless ways are found to prevent and control the adult and childhood obesity epidemic.

FACTORS INFLUENCING OBESITY IN MEXICAN–AMERICAN CHILDREN AND YOUTH

Energy Balance

Obesity is the end result of an energy imbalance, in which overall caloric intake exceeds caloric expenditure. The high and increasing levels of obesity in Mexican–American children and youth would suggest strongly that their energy intake exceeds their energy expenditure and that the imbalance has increased over time. This excess of energy intake over expenditure could be the result of changing dietary patterns favoring an increased intake of higher caloric foods, decreased energy expenditure through limited physical activity, or some combination of both effects.

A number of contextual factors also may influence energy balance. Cultural perceptions of children's ideal body physique by parents may influence child feeding patterns, favoring a robust physique early in life and thereby increasing a child's risk of obesity. Another potential contextual influence on energy balance is the generational status of the child's family, in other words, whether the child's family is the first or second or even a later generation living in the United States. Changes in energy balance in first-generation families may be affected by changes in types and quantity of food available after the families immigrate into the United States as well as by the process of acculturation in dietary preferences. Transition from traditional Mexican diets to American diets likewise may affect second and later generation families as succeeding generations become more acculturated. The insecure employment settings and the environment of poverty in which many Mexican Americans live also may have effects on energy balance by influencing dietary choices, physical activity opportunities, and access to health care.

Finally, it is possible that maternal factors, such as pre-pregnancy obesity, and genetic factors may influence obesity risk. A discussion on the potential impact of these factors on energy balance and obesity risk follows.

Dietary Patterns and Obesity Risk

Data from national surveys indicate an overall increase in daily caloric intake, by approximately 150–200 calories, of American adults from 1971 to 2000 (CDC, 2004). The same trend appears to exist with regard to children—a recent IOM report found that "total calorie intake appears to have increased substantially over the past 25 years for preschool children and adolescent boys and girls, with more modest changes for children ages 6–11 years" (IOM, 2006). However, differences in caloric intake in relation to ethnicity were not defined.

Is the increased prevalence of obesity in Mexican–American children and youth related to the quality of their diets? Large scale dietary intake data to address this question were first provided in the HHANES. An analysis of food frequency demonstrated that Mexican–American children and youth reported eating from the recommended four food groups only 70 percent and 55 percent of the time, respectively (Murphy et al., 1990). Further analysis of these data by foreign-born as well as U.S.-born Mexican

Americans demonstrates that foreign-born Mexican Americans reported eating fruits and vegetables more frequently and eating fewer sugars (NRC/IOM, 1999). Similar findings were seen in NHANES III in adolescents. Those adolescents living in less acculturated homes had less fat, protein, and energy in their diets and more folate (Mazur et al., 2003). Intakes of these nutrients increased with acculturation.

In a study of a nationally representative sample of children, dietary recall on two separate days was used to determine the frequency of fast-food intake. Hispanic children were the least likely to eat fast food as compared with non-Hispanic Whites and African Americans (Bowman et al., 2004). However, once gender, SES, and geographic region were controlled, Hispanic youth were similar in fast-food intake to non-Hispanic Whites. In a U.S. Department of Agriculture study, the diets of children and adolescents were examined using data from NHANES (1999–2000) and a healthy eating index, which measured 10 nutritional components, including the intake of recommended fruits and vegetables and of fat (Basiotis, 2004). This study showed that Mexican Americans overall have a better dietary intake profile than non-Hispanic Whites or Blacks. Furthermore, those born in Mexico had better intake profiles than those born in the United States.

Overall, dietary intake studies suggest that less acculturated children and adults have nutritionally better food intakes with respect to fruits and vegetables, however, as acculturation increases so does fat intake. Therefore, maintaining a traditional diet seems to be an important factor in preventing obesity in Mexican–American children and their families.

Physical Activity and Sedentary Behaviors

Physical activity is the second part of the obesity equation. Data from NHANES III on physical activity and television watching (Andersen et al., 1998) showed that Mexican–American boys and girls reported less physical activity (defined as engaging in three bouts of vigorous activity per week) than non-Hispanic White boys (80.2 percent versus 87.9 percent) and girls (72.6 percent versus 77.1 percent). Mexican-American boys and girls also reported watching more television than non-Hispanic Whites—33.3 percent versus 24.3 percent for boys and 28.3 percent versus 15.6 percent for girls watched more than four hours per day. Watching television is a sedentary activity and occupies time that might otherwise be devoted to more active pursuits. In addition, children are exposed to extensive advertising for high-calorie and low-nutrient foods and beverages (IOM, 2006). More research is needed to better define the television-watching habits of Hispanic and Latino children and youth and to determine how the content of Spanish- and English-language programming impacts their physical activity and dietary behaviors.

Data from the 2002 Youth Media Campaign Longitudinal Survey—a national survey on physical activity—showed that Mexican–American youth are significantly less likely to participate in organized sports than non-Hispanic Whites (25.9 percent versus 46.6 percent) and are somewhat less likely to report (within a seven-day period) participation in free-time play activity (74.6 percent versus 79.3 percent) (Duke et al., 2003). This survey also examined barriers to physical activity and found that Hispanic parents more frequently reported barriers related to transportation issues, a lack of appropriate facilities, expense, a lack of parent time, and a lack of neighborhood safety. However, neighborhood safety was the only barrier that was significantly increased for Hispanic parents when compared with the African–American and non-Hispanic White parents (41.2 percent versus 13.3 percent and 8.5 percent, respectively).

Other data on Hispanic adolescents show similar findings. The California Health Interview Survey 2003 found less regular physical activity among Hispanic (primarily Mexican American) than non-Hispanic White adolescents. Moreover, twice the percentage of Hispanic teens reported no physical activity when compared with non-Hispanic Whites (9.5 percent versus 4.1 percent) (Babey et al., 2005). Only 70 percent of Hispanic teens were in schools that required physical education. In those schools, Hispanic adolescents reported doing regular physical activity significantly more often than Hispanic adolescents in schools where physical education was not required (70.2 percent versus 58.6 percent). Overall, these studies suggest that Mexican–American children and youth are less engaged in regular physical activity than their non-Hispanic counterparts. Barriers to physical activity include the perception of unsafe neighborhoods, the cost (in dollars and time) of sport activities, and the lack of local recreational opportunities such as parks and open spaces. The latter is significant since soccer was reported as the most preferred sport of Hispanic teens in the 2002 Youth Media Campaign Longitudinal Survey.

Culturally Based Perceptions that Influence Obesity

The perception of desirable body physique and what is considered "normal weight" can influence obesity risk by affecting dietary and physical activity behaviors. These perceptions have cultural overlays from current experience (e.g., from the fashion industry) and past experiences such as familial experiences with malnutrition or recurrent illness. These issues need to be explored with Mexican Americans, because they come from a complex cultural milieu involving both Mexican and American influences. Moreover, with a large proportion of immigrants recently arrived from Mexico and the majority of Mexican Americans maintaining some ties to the Latino culture, perceptions of normal weight for Mexican–American children, youth, and parents may be quite different from those of non-Hispanics.

Maynard et al. (2003) examined the NHANES III data to explore maternal perceptions of their children's weight status. Although only 65 percent of mothers identified their children as overweight when they had a BMI greater than the 95th percentile, there was no difference in this ability between Mexican–American and non-Hispanic White mothers (Maynard et al., 2003). However, using the same survey, Klaudt et al. (2002) found that Mexican–American mothers who rated their children as being at the correct weight or at a low weight had children with a higher BMI compared with non-Hispanic White mothers. This finding raises the possiblity that Mexican–American mothers believe that a more rotund physique is normal. Even though the child might not be obese by BMI standards, if the mother's perception is that a "plump" child is healthy, then this perception will need to be addressed so that interventions to control obesity can be successful. Consequently, future research should seek to uncover a better understanding of what Mexican–American mothers consider to be good parenting practices with regard to diet and physical activity.

A more complete understanding of cultural perceptions regarding child rearing may need to involve educating not only the parents but also the entire extended family and community. Familism—the importance of family and culture—is a fundamental factor in Mexican–American families. Romero et al. (2004) hypothesized that this would be strongest in less-educated, Spanish-speaking, and poor families. Instead, the greater levels of familism were seen in those with more education, higher income, and bilingual or English-speaking families. Although this study involved a large, mobile immigrant population, it suggests that even with acculturation, Mexican Americans still retain a strong family orientation. As such, lifestyle changes for Mexican–American children probably will be achieved best by supporting changes at the family and community levels.

Generational Status

Analyses of the HHANES data found that differences in height and weight among immigrant and U.S.-born Mexican–American children were primarily the result of parental SES, and that birthplace did not contribute significantly to either weight or height (NRC/IOM, 1999). Mexican–American children, whether U.S.- or non-U.S. born, had relatively normal weights during childhood compared to their heights. However, during adolescence there was more variability in weights between adolescent boys and girls, particularly with first-generation boys who demonstrated the lowest weights. In HHANES, 12–18-year-old adolescents showed increasing obesity in later generations. However, being foreign born did not demonstrate any difference in BMI for Mexican–American adolescents once age, gender, and SES were controlled (NRC/IOM, 1999). In another study that used data from the National Longitudinal Study of Adolescent Health, Hispanic adolescents born in the United States were twice as likely to be obese than those born outside of the country (Popkin and Udry, 1998). Mexican Americans were the largest Hispanic group in the sample and had the highest percentage (32 percent) over the 85th percentile (considered to be at-risk for obesity). Thus, these studies suggest that U.S.-born Mexican–American youth are more obese than those born in Mexico. This finding is consistent with recent data from the National Health Interview Survey indicating significantly higher rates of obesity and hypertension among U.S.-born Hispanic adults when compared with Hispanic immigrants residing in the United States for less than five years (CDC, 2006).

Acculturation

Acculturation is the process of changing cultural customs, attitudes, perceptions, and behaviors. The time frame of the acculturation process varies from individual to individual and is driven by the living environment and other social pressures for acculturation, such as schools, friends, media, and work. Measures of acculturation usually assess changes in language usage, food preferences, leisure preferences, and social networks. The process of acculturation also can involve changes in perceptions and models of health and well-being that can have a major impact on an individual's health behaviors and assessments of health risk. Even though generational and immigrant status are linked closely to the acculturation process, they are not the same. For that reason, the effects of acculturation on Hispanic obesity need to be explored further.

In a study of immigrant Hispanic adults sampled from the National Health Interview Survey 1998, those who were in the United States for 15 years or longer had a greater likelihood of having a BMI of 30 or greater (Kaplan et al., 2004). Among Hispanics who had been in the United States fewer than 5 years, 9.4 percent had a BMI greater than 30; among those who had been in the United States for more than 15 years, 24.2 percent had a BMI greater than 30. In this study, Mexican Americans were more than 50 percent of the sample and had the highest proportion of obese adults.

In a study conducted in Washington State, Mexican immigrants were found to consume fewer fruits and vegetables as they became more acculturated (Neuhouser et al., 2004). Using data from NHANES III, Dixon et al. (2000) examined the differences in dietary intakes of adult Mexican–American men and women and found that those who were less acculturated took in less fat and more fiber and vitamins. Although these studies focused primarily on adults, they suggest that as immigrants become more acculturrated, their diets change and obesity increases from one generation to the next. Since Mexican–American children and youth comprise such a large proportion of those living in immigrant families, the processes involved in acculturation may be major factors in the increasing prevalence of obesity.

Workforce Participation and the Environment of Poverty

Mexican Americans, who comprise two-thirds of all U.S. Hispanics, continue to be one of the poorest and youngest groups of Americans, with 37 percent of the populations under 18 years of age. The U.S. Census reports that 21.9 percent of Hispanic families live in poverty. In addition, even though Mexican Americans have a workforce participation equal to that of non-Hispanic Whites, they have the highest rate of being uninsured (BLS, 2004; DeNavas-Walt et al., 2005). Both parents typically are working to support their families, a situation that makes child care a major issue. This is particularly true for immigrant families who have higher rates of poverty (Burgos et al., 2005). In addition, with low levels of education, Mexican–American parents tend to have lower paying jobs that are less likely to provide insurance. Their jobs often have less security and typically less union protection, particularly for farm workers before their unionization. Thus, although Mexican Americans have high workforce participation, they continue to live in poverty without health insurance and with limited upward mobility. These realities will impact efforts to prevent obesity by limiting the availability of money to buy healthy food, live in safe areas, and have health insurance to receive preventive and therapeutic medical care.

Though many live in poverty, Mexican Americans are a heterogeneous population in many different ways: economically, culturally, educationally, and even regionally. The status of Mexican Americans currently is undergoing a dramatic change, which can be seen in states like California where Mexican Americans now hold leadership positions in government. This diversity in the population, from the poorest to the most powerful, needs to be considered in developing a strategic plan to improve the problem of obesity in this community while maintaining a focus on those most at risk and least able to help themselves.

Maternal and Genetic Effects on Obesity Risk

Recent studies have suggested that maternal factors such as prepregnancy obesity may influence subsequent obesity risk for children, especially if born to a Hispanic mother (Whitaker, 2004; Salsberry and Reagan, 2005). Genetic factors that may influence energy usage through variable metabolic rates and the degree of fat storage are also potentially important. Preliminary studies in American–Pima Indian populations have shown genotypes in which metabolic rates that are lower by as much as 150 Kcal/d, such that the unburned calories may increase the risk of obesity (Kovacs et al., 2005). The study's investigators were unable to show a direct association with obesity; however, further research may demonstrate a genetic risk for this population that would have significant implications for Mexican Americans who may share the same genotype. Thus, it is possible that Mexican and Mexican–American children with a high proportion of indigenous ancestry may have a greater tendency toward obesity.

CURRENT POLICIES AND PROGRAMS

Various intervention activities have been developed to address child obesity, including media-based health promotion, school-based interventions, community-level activities, health care and family counseling, and research and monitoring. Information on current intervention programs is available from a variety of sources (Action for Healthy Kids, 2005; International Life Sciences Institute, 2005; Shaping America's Youth, 2004). The majority of these interventions have addressed English-speaking audiences, but some programs and materials have been developed in Spanish.

Many current programs have been evaluated to assess their impact on obesity, and the results indicate that the programs have at least short-term reductions in obesity prevalence or improvements in obesity-related dietary and physical activity behaviors. However, these evaluations often are limited methodologically. For example, a recent review of school-based interventions by the Task Force on Community Preventive Services concluded that there was insufficient evidence to determine the effectiveness on children and adolescents of interventions in school settings (CDC, 2005c). Another recent report by the Preventative Services Task Force also cautioned that "interventions to treat overweight adolescents in clinical settings have not been shown to have clinically significant benefits and are not widely available" (Whitlock et al., 2005).

A wide variety of intervention activities that hold promise for successful outcomes are underway although their long-term effectiveness is still to be demonstrated. A number of these interventions have been adapted for use with Spanish-speaking children and families. As noted in the IOM report *Preventing Childhood Obesity: Health in the Balance*, it would be detrimental to wait for conclusive evidence before moving forward with interventions that, based on available evidence, are most likely to provide positive results (IOM, 2005).

This section provides an overview of current intervention activities in the media, schools, communities, and health care settings, as well as related research and monitoring activities. Primary attention is paid to policies and programs that are focused on or relevant to obesity prevention in Mexican–American or other Hispanic children and youth.

Media-Based Health Promotion

The widespread access of Mexican–American families to Spanish media offers promising opportunities to provide health promotion information through media channels. The great majority of Mexican–American families have daily access to television, and radio continues to be a prominent media source for Latinos (Kissam et al., 2003). Access to the Internet is increasing rapidly. Studies by the Pew Internet and American Life Project found that half of all adult Hispanics who speak English had used the Internet and that 78 percent of those with Internet access are online at least 3–5 times a week (Spooner and Rainie, 2001). Although Mexican Americans have substantial media access, the quality of health information disseminated over these channels varies considerably in quality and consistency. Broadie et al. (1999) found that even though Latinos sought out information from the general media, they did not trust the media for health information and felt that media sources did not cover the health issues most relevant to minority communities.

Television viewing by Mexican–American children and youth may be particularly important as both a causal factor in obesity and as a potential source of intervention. A recent IOM report, *Food Marketing to Children and Youth: Threat or Opportunity*, found that children are being exposed to extensive advertising for high-calorie, low-nutrient foods but very limited advertising for more healthful foods and beverages (IOM, 2006). Information on the media exposure of "tweens" and "teens" is available, but there does not appear to be a current content analysis of food and beverage advertisements directed at Hispanic and Latino children and youth despite a high level of expenditure on Hispanic media and advertising (Roberts et al., 2005; Endicott et.al., 2005).

Efforts are underway, however, to improve both the quantity and quality of health information content, although their effectiveness still needs to be evaluated (Velez-Subervi, 1999). Descriptions of some of the more prominent Spanish-language media-based activities initiated by both government and privately sponsored organizations follow. Additional Spanish-language media activities are summarized in tabular form.

Government-Sponsored Media Interventions

Government agencies in the United States and Mexico have initiated media-based interventions to promote healthy eating and physical activity. Some of these programs are briefly described below. Table C-2 summarizes

TABLE C-2 Government-Sponsored Media Interventions

Program	Target Group	Program Description	Evaluation and Contact Information
VERB	"Tweens" (9–13 years)	- Social marketing campaign launched by CDC to promote physical activity. - Uses paid TV and radio advertising. - Website provides information and interactive games to motivate "tweens" and families to be physically active (http://www.verbnow.com/). - Includes health promotion content in Spanish on the CDC website.	- Based on formative research of attitudes and practices of youth relating to physical activity. - At one year, 74 percent of children aware of VERB. - Self-reported physical activity increased. Contact: http://www.cdc.gov/youthcampaign/research/resources.htm http://www.cdc.gov/spanish/VERB/Ninos percent20activos.htm
Eat Smart, Play Hard	6–18 years	- Website displays educational materials in Spanish for use in schools and community programs. - Materials include posters, activity workbooks, brochures, and bookmarks.	- Developed by the U.S. Department of Agriculture Contact: http://www.fns.usda.gov/eatsmartplayhard/Collection/sp-collect_tools.html

information about these programs and provides information about several additional, government-sponsored media intervention activities.

VERB

The VERB campaign was developed by the Centers for Disease Control and Prevention (CDC) as a five-year social marketing campaign for "tweens," children of ages 9–13 years. The campaign is based on formative research that assessed youths' attitudes and practices relating to physical activity. Longitudinal evaluation of the campaign's impact demonstrated

TABLE C-2 Continued

Program	Target Group	Program Description	Evaluation and Contact Information
Todo en Sobrepeso y Obesidad	Older teens and adults	- Provides information on obesity and related cardiovascular risks for patients, health professionals, and families. - Content is culturally and linguistically adapted for use by Mexican Americans. - Related site, Todo en Diabetes, provides information for patients, professionals, and families concerned about diabetes.	Developed by Mexican Government Contact: http://www.todoensalud.org/Obesidad/jsp/intro_fam.jsp http://www.todoensalud.org/diabetes/jsp/Login.jsp
BAM	9–13 years	- Online site developed by CDC. - Provides information to help tweens make healthy behavioral choices.	Contact: http://www.bam.gov/site_terms.html
Powerful Bones, Powerful Girls	Tweens and teenage girls	- Online nutrition and physical activity site developed by CDC and the National Osteoporosis Foundation.	Contact: http://www.cdc.gov/powerfulbones
Small Steps/Kids	Primary school age	- U.S. Department of Health and Human Services health promotion site for kids. - Links to adult site with Spanish content.	Contact: http://www.smallstep.gov/kids/index.cfm

positive effects. Surveys conducted at baseline and at one year after the launch of the campaign found that 74 percent of the children surveyed were aware of the VERB campaign. Levels of self-reported, free-time physical activity increased among various subgroups of children aware of the campaign when compared with levels in children who were unaware of VERB (Huhman et al., 2005). Ongoing evaluation of the VERB campaign will provide valuable information on the potential effectiveness of Web-based health promotion. Though the VERB website for "tweens" does not have Spanish-language content, its images, games, and activities are designed to be appealing to all ethnic groups. VERB has health promotion information in Spanish on the CDC website, with links to a wide variety of health information.

Eat Smart, Play Hard

The U.S. Department of Agriculture (USDA) has also launched a national nutrition education and promotion campaign called Eat Smart, Play Hard, which was targeted at preschool and school-age children and their caregivers. The campaign uses multiple communication vehicles, approaches, and channels, including print materials and the Internet. In addition to English-language content, the campaign's website displays Spanish-language educational materials designed for use by children and adolescents in schools and community programs.

Todo en Sobrepeso y Obesidad

The Mexican government, in collaboration with professional societies and industry partners, has developed a health information website: Todo En Sobrepeso y Obesidad. The site provides information on obesity and related cardiovascular risks for patients, health professionals, and families. Because it originates in Mexico, the content is culturally and linguistically adapted for use by Mexican Americans. A related site, Todo en Diabetes, provides information specifically for patients, professionals, and families concerned about or caring for persons with diabetes.

Privately-Sponsored Media Interventions

A variety of media-based interventions also have been privately sponsored. Some of the more prominent programs that provide Spanish-language content follow. These programs also are summarized in Table C-3, along with several additional privately supported media interventions.

Salud es Vida . . . Enterate!

Television and radio broadcasters have potential to reach a great number of Hispanics with health information. A prominent example is the health education initiative of Univision Communications Inc., Salud es Vida . . . Enterate!, which was launched in 2003. This health promotion effort provides informational messages and programming—including public service announcements (PSAs), vignettes, news, and dedicated health programs featuring nationally recognized Hispanic celebrities and medical experts—on radio and television. To complement this effort, Univision.com has developed a comprehensive Spanish-language website that provides information

TABLE C-3 Privately Sponsored Media Interventions

Program	Target Group	Program Description	Evaluation and Contact Information
Salud es Vida . . . Enterate!!	Parents and Older teens	- Sponsored by Univision. - Television and radio: Provides informational messages and programming on radio and television including PSAs, vignettes, news, and dedicated health programs. - Internet: Interactive website provides information on health issues and advice on healthful nutrition and physical activities. - Partners with Univision in this initiative include the Kaiser Family Foundation, the Ad Council, and many other health, community, and medical organizations.	- Impact evaluated based on calls to the Spanish-language call center of the American Diabetes Association. Contact: Univision Communications Inc. http://www.univision.com/content/channel.jhtml?chid=2&schid=8241 http://www.kff.org/entpartnerships/Univision-Announces-Year-Long-Health-Campaign-in-Partnership-With-the-Kaiser-Family-Foundation.cfm
Coalition for Healthy Children	Children, teens, and parents	- Involves marketers, media, nonprofits, foundations, and government agencies to provide consistent, research-based messages targeted to parents and children. - Coalition members incorporate messages into their communications activities. - Use of key messages to be reported by participating organizations to the Ad Council and shared with Coalition members via an online forum.	- Program impact to be measured by changes in attitudes and behavior of children and parents. - Results to be published and distributed to key constituencies. - No specific plans for translation into Spanish, but coalition members could address this need and share their efforts with others. Contact: http://healthychildren.adcouncil.org/about.asp
Kidnetic	Primary school kids and teens	- Physical activity and nutrition promotion site developed by the International Food Information Council.	Contact: http://kidnetic.com/Whatis.aspx

continued

TABLE C-3 Continued

Program	Target Group	Program Description	Evaluation and Contact Information
Shaping America's Youth	All ages	- Online resource listing obesity programs. - Sponsors include Cadbury, Schweppes, Campbell Soup, FedEx, NIKE.	Contact: http://www.shaping americas youth. org/ Default.aspx

on a wide range of health issues and advice on healthful nutrition and physical activities. The campaign is not directed at children or adolescents, but the messages do reach Hispanic parents who are seeking information about nutrition, physical activity, and being overweight as those topics relate to caring for their children. Partners with Univision in this initiative include the Kaiser Family Foundation, the Ad Council, the American Diabetes Association and many other health, community, and medical organizations.

Coalition for Healthy Children: Combating Childhood Obesity

Another initiative to enhance health information for children and youth is the Coalition for Healthy Children, a public–private collaboration designed to use the collective strengths of marketers, the media, nonprofits, foundations, and government agencies to address the obesity crisis. With support from the Robert Wood Johnson Foundation and in cooperation with the Advertising Council, the coalition aims to provide consistent, research-based messages targeted at parents and children. The coalition's strategy is to have each of its members incorporate these common messages into their communications activities, including advertising, packaging, websites, grassroots programs, and marketing events. Program impact will be assessed through an ongoing tracking study. Although no specific plans have been developed for translating these or other messages into Spanish, coalition members could address this need and share their efforts with others.

School-Based Interventions

A wide variety of school-based intervention programs have been developed but few are designed specifically for Hispanic children. However, Spanish-language teaching materials are available from a number of sources, and many programs and policies that promote physical activity and provide for healthful food choices in schools can benefit all children, including Mexican Americans.

Implementing school-based obesity interventions can present a number of challenges (GAO, 2005). Changes in school curriculum to include more nutrition education or increased physical activity opportunities must be integrated into and contend with other academic priorities. Physical activity programs may be less controversial since changes in school food or vending policies must deal with the added costs of providing more healthful meals and possible lost income from vending contracts. School administrators cite a lack of program models and clear guidelines but at the same time want flexibility to adapt interventions to meet their local needs and resources.

Despite these challenges, many school-based interventions have been initiated (Food and Nutrition Service, 2005). Several intervention programs, including Bienestar and CATCH, have been undertaken and evaluated in schools with a high proportion of Mexican–American children. These intervention programs have combined nutrition education and have increased opportunities for physical activity with policy changes with regard to vending and the nutritional quality of school meals. These programs provide examples of promising strategies for school-based intervention that have been successful in schools with a high proportion of Mexican–American children. A complementary strategy, described below, is the development of school wellness policies as required by recent federal legislation. Finally, Table 4-3 lists resources for obtaining Spanish-language educational materials for classroom instruction and for sharing with parents, although the effectiveness of these materials has not been evaluated.

Bienestar

Developed in San Antonio, Texas, Bienestar is a bilingual, nutrition and physical activity promotion program designed specifically for use in elementary schools with a high proportion of Hispanic children. The intervention is based on social cognitive theory that recognizes the need to change the social systems that influence children's behaviors. In line with this theoretical construct, the intervention consists of programs targeting parents, school health classes, cafeterias, and after-school programs.

The impact of the intervention on obesity and diabetes risk factors was evaluated, and the results were reported in a recent study in San Antonio, Texas (Trevino et al., 2005). This randomized, controlled trial found that after adjusting for covariates the mean fasting capillary glucose levels decreased in the intervention schools and increased in control schools. Fitness scores increased significantly in intervention children and decreased in control children. However, no significant difference was found in the percentage of body fat. Even though longer follow-up will be needed to determine long-term benefits, these results indicate the potential success of a multi-component, bilingual intervention to modify risk factors for diabetes.

CATCH

The Coordinated Approach to Child Health (CATCH) program in El Paso, Texas, implemented a school-based intervention to increase moderate to vigorous physical activity and to improve the nutritional content of school meals. Evaluation in 24 schools with a high proportion of Mexican–American children found that, for most intervention schools, the intervention was associated with significantly increased moderate to vigorous physical activity and decreased fat in school meals. However, some schools did not meet fat content goals, and no schools met the vigorous physical activity goals (Heath and Coleman, 2002). Other follow-up studies in a cohort of children from ethnically diverse backgrounds in California, Louisiana, Minnesota, and Texas have shown that behavioral changes associated with the CATCH intervention were maintained for three years without further intervention. Although not specific to any single ethnic group, these findings suggest that behavioral changes initiated during the elementary school years may persist into early adolescence (Nader et al., 1999).

Wellness Policy Development

An important policy development stemming from the Child Nutrition and WIC (Special Supplemental Nutrition Program for Women, Infants, and Children) Reauthorization Act of 2004 requires all school districts with a federally-funded school meals program to develop and implement wellness policies that address nutrition and physical activity by the start of the 2006–2007 school year. This new requirement for a defined wellness policy presents a significant opportunity for advancing school-based nutrition and physical activity promotion. School administrators, teachers, and parents should be encouraged to use the opportunity to review current policies and identify changes that can improve the healthfulness of the school environment and contribute to obesity prevention.

A number of resources are available to assist schools in developing wellness policies. The National Alliance for Nutrition and Activity has developed a set of model policies for use by local school districts. Resources to aid schools in formulating wellness policies include CDC's School Health Index, USDA's Changing the Scene guidelines, and wellness policy development tools trainings from Action for Healthy Kids (Table C-4). Support for developing and implementing school wellness policies should be a high priority.

TABLE C-4 School-Based Interventions and Teaching Materials

Program	Target Group	Program Description	Evaluation and Contact Information
Bienestar	Grades 3–5	- Bilingual instructional material. - Intervention based on social cognitive theory. - Programs target parents, school health classes, cafeterias, and after-school activities. - Primary objectives are to decrease dietary fat intake, increase fiber intake, increase physical fitness, and control body weight.	- Randomized controlled trial results show that intervention students have • Significantly increased dietary fiber intake, • Increased physical fitness levels, and • Decreased fasting capillary glucose levels. - However, no significant difference was found in the percentage of body fat in intervention and control children (Trevino et al., 2005). Contact: Social and Health Research Center http://www.sahrc.org/
CATCH (Coordinated Approach to Child Health)	Intervene grades K–5 Follow-up grades 6–8	Environmental Change Goals: - Reduce total fat, saturated fat, and sodium content of food served in school meals. - Increase the percent of physical education class time that students spend in moderate to vigorous physical activity to 40 percent. - CATCH Kids Club After School Program is available: http://www.flaghouse.com/afterSchool.asp	- Evaluation in 24 schools with a high proportion of Mexican–American children. - Intervention associated with significantly increased moderate to vigorous physical activity and decreased fat in school meals. - However, some schools did not meet fat content goals, and no schools met vigorous physical activity goals (Heath and Coleman, 2002). Contact: http://www.flaghouse.com/CatchPE.asp

continued

TABLE C-4 Continued

Program	Target Group	Program Description	Evaluation and Contact Information
School Wellness Policy Development	School staff and parents	- National Alliance for Nutrition and Activity (NANA) offers guidance on developing school wellness policies and lists resources from CDC and USDA. - Action for Healthy Kids also provides online guidelines.	Contact: http://www.schoolwellnesspolicies.org/ http://apps.nccd.cdc.gov/shi/default.aspx http://www.fns.usda.gov/tn/Healthy/changing.html http://www.actionforhealthykids.org/resources_wp.php
My Pyramid for Kids	Grades K–5	- Spanish version of USDA's "My Pyramid" food and physical activity guide.	Contact: http://teamnutrition.usda.gov/kids-pyramid.html
MiPirámide	Children and teens	- A Spanish-language version of MyPyramid.gov. MiPirámide: Pasos Hacia Una Mejor Salud, MyPyramid: Steps to a Healthier You emphasizes the same key messages as MyPyramid: • Making smart choices from every food group, • Finding a balance between food intake and physical activity, and • Getting the most nutrition from calories consumed.	- The MyPyramid graphics, website, and handouts and other materials have been translated into Spanish. These resources can be accessed at http://www.MyPyramid.gov.
What's to Eat	Parents and older children	- Spanish version of a video to assist families prepare and enjoy healthy food. - Stanford Health Promotion Resource Center	Contact: http://hprc.stanford.edu/pages/store/catalog.asp?Spanish
Learning Zone Express	Grades K–12	- Posters and teaching aids in Spanish. - Online store and resource center.	Contact: http://www.learningzoneexpress.com

Community-Based Interventions

Many community level interventions have been initiated to promote physical activity and nutrition improvement in children, adolescents, and adults. Examples of programs that specifically address the needs of Hispanic children and youth are described in the following sections as are more general programs that assist the community as a whole in implementing obesity prevention strategies. The programs cited are summarized in Table C-5.

Government-Sponsored Interventions

Diviértase y Sea Activo

Diviértase y Sea Activo (Have Fun and Be Active) is the title of a physical activity program funded by the Contra Costa Children and Families Commission of Contra Costa County, California. A video, available in Spanish and English, encourages families to choose a healthy, active lifestyle by showing images of families participating in variety of physical activities. A related activity also provided by the Commission is the scheduling of community health promotion fairs for Hispanic families; the fairs are advertised to the community as Diviértase y Manténgase Saludable Talleres (Have Fun and Be Healthy Workshops). At these events families learn to prepare healthy snacks, play games, and participate in fun physical activities. This program provides an interesting model in which activities potentially contributing to obesity prevention can be integrated into a larger framework of community efforts to promote child health.

California Latino 5-a-Day

California's Latino 5-a-Day program promotes fruit and vegetable consumption among Spanish-speaking adults. The intervention is designed to reach Latinos in their homes, where they shop, where they eat, and where they gather with other community members. Evaluation of the program's impact by telephone interviews found a significant increase in fruit and vegetable consumption and increased awareness of the 5-a-Day message among Spanish-speakers in the target area of the campaign. Although the program does not directly address children and adolescents, the campaign may have an impact by modifying parent's attitudes and food purchase behaviors. California also has developed a Children's 5-a-Day Power Play Campaign targeted to 9–11-year-old children. Even though the program is not presented in Spanish, it is designed to appeal to English-speaking Latino children.

TABLE C-5 Government-Sponsored Interventions

Program	Target Group	Program Description	Evaluation and Contact Information
Diviértase y Sea Activo	1–5 years	- An initiative of the Contra Costa Children and Families Commission that includes the following: • Video, in Spanish, showing families being physically active with children ages 1–5 years. • Community health promotion fairs for Hispanic families.	Contact for purchase of the video: http://www.abridgeclub.com/Videos_&_DVD.htm#Have%20Fun%20&%20Be%20Active Brochure for health fair: http://www.cchealth.org/espanol/pdf/wic_funshops_esp_2005_10.pdf
California Latino 5-a-Day Children's 5-a-Day Power Play		- Promotes fruit and vegetable consumption among Spanish-speaking adults. - Designed to reach Latinos in their homes and communities. - Have developed Children's 5-a-Day Power Play Campaign targeted to 9–11-year-old children. - Not in Spanish but designed to appeal to Latino children who speak English.	- Evaluation by telephone interviews found an increase in fruit and vegetable consumption and increased awareness of the 5-a-Day message among Spanish-speakers. - Not addressing children and adolescents directly, but may have impact by modifying parents' attitudes and food purchases. Contact: http://www.dhs.ca.gov/ps/cdic/cpns/lat5aday/lat_research.htm
Food Stamp Program		- Assists low-income families in buying nutritious foods. - Eligibility based on income; all children born in the United States are entitled to the benefits. - However, many eligible Latinos do not participate in the program.	Contact: http://www.sfgate.com/cgi-bin/article.cgi?file=/chronicle/archive/2004/10/01/BAGG691K4B1.DTL

Food Stamp Program

Participation in the food stamp program can assist low-income families in buying nutritious foods that may be less likely to contribute to obesity. Eligibility for food stamps is based on income, and all children born in the United States are entitled to the benefits. However, a survey by the Alameda County Community Food Bank estimated that 1.7 million Californians, many of them Latino, are eligible for food stamps but do not participate in the program. These findings suggest that an educational campaign to expand awareness of and participation in the food stamp program by Mexican Americans could help improve access to healthful foods and would be a valuable component of an overall obesity prevention strategy.

Private and Community-Sponsored Interventions

Many promising community-based programs have been initiated by private and non-profit organizations that are concerned with the health and welfare of children. Examples of such programs are described in the following sections and summarized in Table C-6.

CANFit

The California Adolescent Nutrition and Fitness (CANFit) Program is designed to help communities build the capacity to improve the nutrition and physical activity status of low-income ethnic youth who are 10–14 years old. CANFit has launched health promotion campaigns specifically addressing the Hispanic community. For example, the Adelante con Leche Semi-descremada 1 percent campaign, implemented in Los Angeles in 1999–2000, was designed to motivate Latino youth and their families to switch from drinking whole or two-percent milk, to drinking one-percent or fat-free milk. Based on sales report data, the Adelante campaign resulted in a 200-percent increase in one-percent milk sales (see Table C-6 for reference).

Latino Health Access

Latino Health Access is a community-based health promotion program that uses community health promoters who are recruited to work in the communities where they live. The *promotores* are skilled at educating and serving as role models for their peers. The Children and Youth Initiative, a program of Latino Health Access in California, is a school and community based intervention that is designed specifically for assisting children who

TABLE C-6 Private and Community-Sponsored Interventions

Program	Target Group	Program Description	Evaluation and Contact Information
CANFit (California Adolescent Nutrition and Fitness program)	10–14 years	- Provides training and technical assistance to youth-serving organizations. - Develops educational materials and social marketing programs. - Advocates for policies that enhance nutrition and physical activity. - Awards academic scholarships. - Funds innovative community-based projects. - CANFit is funded by private donations.	- Example program: The *Adelante con Leche Semi-descremada 1 percent* campaign. - Promoted switching to one-percent or fat-free milk. - Used paid Hispanic radio, print advertising, and television; one-percent milk tastings. - Resulted in a 200-percent increase in one-percent milk sales. Contact: http://www.canfit.org/programs.html
Latino Health Access	Children and youth	- Uses community health promoters to work in the communities where they live. - *Promotores* are skilled at educating and serving as role models for their peers. - The Children and Youth Initiative assists children in high-risk environments to adopt healthful nutrition and physical activity and other positive behaviors that promote good health.	Contact: http://www.latinohealthaccess.org/aboutus.shtml
Kraft Salsa, Sabor y Salud	Latino families	- An eight-session healthy-lifestyle course for Latino families to reduce risks for obesity and related health problems. - Since 2003, the program has reached nearly 10,000 adults and children in 50 community organizations in six states.	Contact: http://www.kraft.com/responsibility/nhw_communitybased.aspx

TABLE C-6 Continued

Program	Target Group	Program Description	Evaluation and Contact Information
Latino Nutrition Coalition	Latino families	- A consortium of industry, scientists and chefs in collaboration with the Oldways Preservation Trust. - Promotes programs in food stores, schools, restaurants, and clinics and sponsors community events.	Contact: http://www.latinonutrition.org/ http://oldwayspt.org/index.php?area=latino_nutrition_coalition

live in high-risk environments to adopt nutrition, physical activity, and other positive behaviors that promote good health.

Salsa, Sabor y Salud

Kraft has partnered with the National Latino Children's Institute to develop Salsa, Sabor y Salud (Food, Fun, and Fitness), an eight-session healthy-lifestyle course for Latino families. The program supports Hispanic families in adopting healthy lifestyles that will reduce the risk of obesity and related health problems. Launched in 2003, Salsa, Sabor y Salud has reached nearly 10,000 adults and children through 50 community organizations in six states.

Latino Nutrition Coalition

The Latino Nutrition Coalition is a consortium of industry leaders, scientists, and chefs in cooperation with the Oldways Preservation Trust to promote better Latino health through traditional foods and lifestyles. The Coalition will focus on practical programs of education and promotion in grocery stores, schools, health clinics, and restaurants. Initiatives that will include community fiestas and festivals are planned in five or six cities.

Health Care Interventions

Mexican Americans and other Hispanics face a number of barriers in accessing health care, including language barriers, cultural differences, poverty, lack of health insurance, and transportation difficulties. These challenges complicate the provision of healthcare interventions to prevent and manage obesity in Mexican–American children. Evaluation of interventions in the health care setting has encountered methodological limitations. In 2002 the U.S. Preventive Services Task Force concluded that "the evidence is insufficient to recommend for or against behavioral counseling in primary care settings to promote physical activity," noting that there were no completed trials with children or adolescents that compared counseling with usual care practices (USPSTF, 2002). In 2003 another task force report concluded that "the evidence is insufficient to recommend for or against routine behavioral counseling to promote a healthy diet in unselected patients in primary care settings," noting that "no controlled trials of routine behavioral dietary counseling for children or adolescents in the primary care setting were identified" (USPSTF, 2003). As noted previously, a recent task force report cautioned that "interventions to treat overweight adolescents in clinical settings have not been shown to have clinically significant benefits and are not widely available." Although much more needs to be done to provide a more adequate research base, both government-sponsored and privately supported efforts are underway to address obesity in clinical settings. Examples of health care interventions that address Hispanic populations are highlighted in the following sections and are summarized in Table 4-6.

Government-Supported Health Care Interventions

Vida Saludable, Corazon Contento

The *Vida Saludable, Corazon Contento* guide is translated and adapted from the WISEWOMAN CVD prevention program for underserved and underinsured women ages 40 to 64 years. Funded by CDC, this program offers guidance to health care providers on screening for CVD risk factors, lifestyle counseling to improve diet and physical activity, and clinical referral and follow-up services. The program involves a three-session intervention that emphasizes readiness for change, goal-setting, individual tailoring, self-monitoring, and social support. Counseling is facilitated by bilingual community health workers. Although not designed to reach children and adolescents directly, the information and support provided to Spanish-speaking women potentially can assist in promoting healthy dietary and physical activity practices within their families. California currently is planning to pilot test the guide in five sites.

WIC Program

The WIC program serves 8 million women, infants, and children—almost half of the United States' infants and a quarter of 1–5 year olds. In 2002, for the first time, Hispanics made up the largest group of WIC participants (38.1 percent) (Table C-7). In states with a high proportion of Latinos, the great majority of WIC participants are Latino. For example, in California, 70 percent of WIC participants are Latino. This high level of participation makes the WIC program a major point of contact for Latinos with health care professionals and an important potential source of counseling with regard to a healthful diet and physical activity. At the same time, the limitations of the WIC program are clear: the program provides only limited health counseling on an infrequent basis. Such minimal exposure and follow-up is unlikely to be adequate to substantially affect behaviors.

Privately Sponsored Healthcare Interventions

The Kidshape family lifestyle intervention is designed to promote healthful dietary and physical activity behaviors in 6–14-year-old overweight children and their parents. This clinical intervention has been implemented in various locations in southern California. The program is now being implemented in both English and Spanish in a clinic in northern California (Contra Costa County) as part of a larger community-based effort to prevent and treat childhood obesity in a population with a high proportion of Mexican Americans. The eight-week program is family oriented and requires that both parents and children attend all of the weekly sessions. It is reported that 87 percent of children lose weight and 80 percent maintain weight loss 1.5–2.5 years after finishing the program, but the Kidshape website does not provide the supporting data (Table C-7). While clearly needing evaluation, the Kidshape program is an example of the type of family-based clinical intervention that seems most promising.

Research and Monitoring

Research and monitoring activities are a critical part of the overall strategy to prevent child obesity. As noted above, there are intrinsic challenges in conducting evaluations of school-based and community intervention programs. Continuing and expanded research is needed to define best practices and demonstrate effectiveness. Ongoing monitoring of weight status and behavioral trends also is needed to gauge long-term progress in obesity prevention.

TABLE C-7 Government-Supported and Privately Sponsored Health Care Interventions

Program	Target Group	Program Description	Evaluation and Contact Information
Vida Saludable, Corazon Contento	Women 40–64 years	- Translated and adapted from the WISEWOMAN CVD prevention program funded by CDC. - Offers guidance to health care providers in screening for CVD risk factors, lifestyle counseling to improve diet and physical activity, and clinical referral and follow-up services. - Support provided to Spanish-speaking women to promote healthy diet and physical activity within their families.	- The three-session intervention emphasizes readiness for change, goal-setting, individual tailoring, self-monitoring, and social support. - Counseling is facilitated by bilingual community health workers. - California is currently planning to pilot test the guide in five sites. Contact: http://www.hpdp.unc.edu/wisewoman/vida.htm http://wwwtest.cdc.gov/wisewoman/project_locations/california.htm
WIC Program	Birth to 5 years	- The WIC program serves 8 million women, infants, and children, almost half of United States' infants and a quarter of children 1–5 years of age. - In 2002, for the first time, Hispanics made up the largest group of WIC participants (38.1). - In California, 70 percent of WIC participants are Latino. - The WIC program is a major point of contact of Latinos with health care professionals.	Contact: http://www.fns.usda.gov/oane/MENU/Published/WIC/FILES/PC2002.htm

TABLE C-7 Continued

Program	Target Group	Program Description	Evaluation and Contact Information
Kidshape	6–14 years and parents	- Offered in Spanish or English. - Eight weekly classes, two hours each. - Parents and children must attend. - Classes focus on healthy eating, behavior change principles, and physical activity.	- Website reports that: • 87 percent lose weight. • 80 percent report sustained weight loss at 1.5–2.5 year follow-up. Contact: http://www.cchealth.org/espanol/detalles_sobre_kidshape.html http://www.kidshape.com/Pages/programs.htm

National-Level Survey and Monitoring Activities

At the national level in the United States, the ongoing Health and Nutrition Examination surveys, Behavioral Risk Factor Surveillance surveys, and Youth Risk Behavior surveys provide essential information on obesity prevalence and behavioral trends. However, data from these sources may not be specific or detailed enough to characterize and monitor the attitudes and behaviors of children and youth with regard to dietary and physical activity behaviors. To address this need, CDC has developed the Youth Media Campaign Longitudinal Survey (YMCLS), an annual national telephone survey of young people ages 9–13 years and their parents. The YMCLS is designed to measure the physical activity–related beliefs, attitudes, and behaviors of youth and their parents and to monitor youth exposure to the VERB social marketing campaign. Survey results provide information on the VERB campaign's impact and guide the campaign's evolution.

The surveys also provide a valuable research base that can aid in the design of other obesity prevention efforts. More specifically, focused interviews with Hispanic teens and parents documented a variety of cultural attitudes that may affect the adoption of healthful physical activity behaviors (Table C-8). For example, Hispanic youth are encouraged to put family needs above their own, and activity for personal benefit may be discouraged. Household chores and baby-sitting younger siblings after school while parents work were identified as barriers, especially for girls. Physical activ-

TABLE C-8 Research and Monitoring Activities

Program	Target Group	Program Description	Evaluation and Contact Information
Youth Media Campaign Longitudinal Survey	9–13 years	- Annual national telephone survey of young people ages 9–13 years and their parents. - Conducted by CDC. - Measures physical activity–related beliefs, attitudes, and behaviors of youth and their parents. - Monitors youth exposure to the VERB campaign. - Evaluates the VERB campaign's impact. - Supplemental interviews with Hispanics provided culture-specific insights.	Contact: http://www.cdc.gov/youthcampaign/research/PDF/4.4.10-HisLatExSummaryRes.pdf
Children's Healthy Eating and Exercise Practices Survey	9–11 years	- Designed to assess dietary and physical activity patterns in children 9–11 years. - Sample of children from 2000 households included 38 percent Latino.	- California Department of Health Services Contact: http://www.dhs.ca.gov/ps/cdic/cpns/research/calcheeps2003.html
Teen Eating, Exercise, and Nutrition Survey	12–17 years	- Provides information on teen dietary and exercise behaviors in 1998. - Assesses differences in behaviors in relation to age and gender.	Contact: http://www.dhs.ca.gov/ps/cdic/cpns/research/calteens2000.html
High School Fast Food Survey		- Conducted in 2003. - Survey examined school food service practices in a sample of California high schools.	- Public Health Institute, 2003 Contact: http://www.phi.org/pdf-library/fastfoodsurvey2000.pdf
California Health Interview Survey	1–18 years	- Conducted in 2001, 2003, 2005 by random dialed telephone survey in multiple languages. - Direct data from adolescents and for children from most knowledgeable adults.	- UCLA Center for Health Policy, School of Public Health Contact: http://www.chis.ucla.edu/default.asp

ity was considered as merely playing and a distraction, and no connection was seen between physical activity and health benefits. Parents were reluctant to involve their kids in programs that didn't seem culturally relevant or that were not sanctioned by cultural authority figures they trust. These data indicate the very useful information obtainable by telephone surveys and supplemental interviews with Hispanic respondents.

State-Level Survey Activities

National data from the sources described previously often are inadequate to assess the status of state populations or specific subgroups that may vary substantially from overall national trends. State- and population-specific surveys frequently are needed to sufficiently assess obesity prevalence and the attitudes and behaviors related to obesity risk. Several California state-level surveillance and monitoring programs that may serve as useful examples are summarized in Table C-8. In particular, the California Health Interview Survey (CHIS)—conducted in English, Spanish, Chinese, Korean, and Vietnamese— is perhaps the nation's most culturally inclusive survey. The CHIS has been used to report on several factors relating to childhood obesity, including dietary intakes, physical activity, and environmental issues contributing to obesity.

Online Formative Research

For Mexican–American parents and youth, having access to the Internet offers the potential to do online research that can reach thousands of respondents. Data provided online are already in electronic form and are ready to be tabulated and analyzed statistically. Respondents provide demographic information such as age, gender, place of residence, income, and education level for use in interpreting the information. Longitudinal follow-up is feasible via e-mail to assess response to an intervention. Research and monitoring using the Internet should be explored as a promising option for future development and evaluation of obesity prevention efforts.

THEORETICAL FRAMEWORK FOR INTERVENTION

Although interventions to treat obesity in children and adolescents who are already overweight can be successful, the process often requires intensive and sustained intervention, and long-term success is not assured. Moreover, Mexican–American children have limited access to health care and costs, and language and other barriers can be significant. These realities underscore the conclusion of the IOM report *Preventing Obesity: Health in the Balance* that the strategy to address childhood obesity must be to focus on primary prevention (IOM, 2005).

A recent series of meetings coordinated by the Berkeley Media Studies Group looked at ways to accelerate the development of effective policies to foster healthier nutrition and eating environments. The "acceleration" meetings reviewed the experience of other public health prevention efforts such as those addressing tobacco, alcohol, firearms, and traffic safety. The summary of these meetings suggested that based on the experience of these other public health efforts the path of least resistance for obesity prevention would be to focus on individual behavior change (Dorfman et al., 2005). This strategy puts the onus of responsibility on individuals to adopt healthful nutrition and physical activity habits. However, individual behavior change is unlikely to be successful unless positive behavioral changes are supported by the media, school, community, and health care environments in which individuals live.

The discussions at the acceleration meetings led to the conclusion that prevention efforts must shift focus from behavior to policy changes that affect the environments where behaviors take place. Although policy changes are more likely to meet more resistance than interventions that focus on individual behavior change, a policy change strategy offers the best opportunity to achieve effective and sustained prevention.

Behavioral Theory

The theoretical framework described in the IOM report *Preventing Obesity: Health in the Balance* used an ecological systems theory model that depicts the behavioral settings and leverage points that influence food intake and energy expenditure (IOM, 2005). The child or adolescent is seen as being at the center of concentric rings of influence from family, school, community, industry, and government, and the larger culture and society. Leverage points that influence behavior include the food system, opportunities for physical activity or sedentary behavior, and information regarding the health implications of dietary behaviors and physical activity. Behavioral choices within this ecological system also are seen as affected by social norms and values.

Another behavioral theory that has been used in conceptualizing strategies for obesity prevention is social learning theory. This theory emphasizes the importance of observing and modeling the behaviors, attitudes, and emotional reactions of others. In this model, developed principally by Bandura, most human behavior is learned through observation and modeling. The social learning theory model, later renamed by Bandura as social cognitive theory, was used in developing the multicomponent, school-based Bienestar intervention (Bandura, 1986; Trevino et al., 1998). According to this model, social systems in the individual's environment, in addition to internal standards and self-evaluation, mediate the relationship between the individual's knowledge and his or her consequent behaviors. Because of the importance of social systems in the individual's environment, the Bienestar program designed components that affected the child's environment in the classroom, cafeteria, after-school, and home settings. Another intervention focusing on increasing fruit and vegetable consumption also used social learning theory by emphasizing changes in the home environment and parental support to achieve positive behavioral changes in 10–12-year-old children (Gribble et al., 2003).

The ecological systems model and the social cognitive theory model both appear to be valid constructs for the development of obesity prevention interventions, since both recognize the importance of environmental factors in influencing behaviors. However, an issue to be considered in using either model is whether Mexican–American families have the same level of empowerment as non-Hispanic families to make changes in schools and community environments. Mexican Americans may be more fatalistic about health or about their ability to make changes. Given these concerns, it is unclear that there currently exists a best practice model for obesity prevention in Mexican–American children. Further research is needed to clarify the kinds of intervention strategies that will work best in Hispanic communities.

Evidence-Based Approach

The IOM report describes the need for an evidence-based approach to the development of obesity prevention interventions by using multiple sources of evidence, including randomized controlled trials (if available), quasi-experimental, and observational studies. It is critical to systematically evaluate the effectiveness of intervention efforts, while at the same time to recognize the practical realities and the fiscal and socio-political environments in which programs are implemented. Because of these constraints, research has evaluated only a limited number of interventions relevant to obesity prevention in Mexican–American children. Additional research is needed to define best practice models in media, school, community, and health care settings. Attention should be focused on the development and testing of community empowerment models and on interventions that draw on and incorporate values and beliefs stemming from Mexican culture, music, art, and literature.

RECOMMENDATIONS FOR ACTION

Overall goals for obesity prevention in Mexican–American children parallel those for all children and youth as expressed in IOM's *Preventing Obesity, Health in the Balance*. In the long term, the overriding goals are to achieve a reduction in the incidence and prevalence of obesity; improve dietary patterns to be consistent with dietary guidelines; meet physical activity guidelines; and achieve physical, psychological, and cognitive growth and development goals. However, more specific intermediate goals and recommendations that address the specific needs of Mexican–American children and youth must be defined.

Achieving policy, environmental, and behavioral goals for obesity prevention for Mexican–American children and youth will require interventions at many levels, including television, print, and electronic media; schools; communities; and health care settings. To be successful, these efforts must be supported by ongoing research and monitoring and by effective advocacy.

Some key issues to be addressed include the following: (a) the need for comprehensive, multifaceted interventions that can address dietary and physical activity behaviors; (b) greater insight into the feasibility of scaling up interventions to programs in large populations groups; and (c) an increased understanding of ways to sustain interventions after initial start-up funds are no longer available. Outlined below are a variety of potential actions that might be recommended and prioritized based on the discussions in the workshop.

Media-Based Interventions

Media-based interventions are appealing because of their potential to reach large target audiences and for their low cost. Given the high level of access that Mexican–American families have to television and radio as well as the growing access they have to the Internet, especially by older children and youth, these media channels are an increasingly important means of providing information and motivation for healthy lifestyle choices. Another appealing feature of media-based interventions is the ability of electronic content to be shared internationally, in particular between Mexico and the Mexican–American populations in the United States. At the same time, food and beverage advertising through the same media can promote consumption of high-calorie and low-nutrient food and beverages and can negatively influence dietary and physical activity behaviors, thus increasing the risk of obesity. Specific actions that support expanding the potential and reducing the negative impact of media-based messages are cited in the following list.

Health Information in Television, Radio, and Print Media

- Establish policies and guidelines that define appropriate marketing of foods and beverages to children and youth in general and specifically to Mexican–American children and youth.

• Increase the number of new industry products and advertising messages that promote energy balance at a healthy weight and are targeted to Mexican–American consumers.

Internet-Based Health Promotion Resources

• Develop culturally appropriate Web content that specifically targets Mexican–American children, youth, and parents.

• Develop Web content in Spanish, or adapt it from existing English language websites, to provide accurate and appealing health information and to offer tips and guidance in choosing healthy lifestyles.

School-Based Interventions

School environments provide an important influence on children's behaviors and can foster healthful nutrition and physical activity or negatively influence these behaviors. Many of the interventions currently being implemented and evaluated are carried out in the school setting. Some key strategies for fostering health-promoting school environments include the following:

• Provide training for and support development of school wellness policies that promote healthful school nutrition and physical activity environments.

• Implement school food service and vending policies that encourage healthful dietary choices.

• Support the development and dissemination of language and culturally appropriate health education materials for Mexican–American children and youth.

• Support research to develop and evaluate school-based interventions that are sustainable and effective in promoting increased participation in healthful physical activity.

Community-Based Interventions

Community-based youth programs and policies that create environments where children, youth, and families can share physical activity are critical components of an obesity prevention strategy.

• Support expansion of community-based youth programs that serve Mexican–American children and youth.

• In neighborhoods with a high proportion of Hispanic families, support policies such as the expansion of park facilities, sidewalks, and bike paths that encourage safe physical activity.

- Provide training opportunities and materials to youth program staff to enhance their effectiveness.
- Give recognition for achievements in developing successful community-based programs that serve Mexican–American populations.
- Improve access to and affordability of fruits and vegetables for low-income Mexican–American populations.
- Encourage participation by Mexican–American families in federal food assistance programs that increase access to healthful foods.
- Implement policies that promote neighborhood safety, improved air quality, public transportation, and design conducive to healthy activity.

Health Care Interventions

Although many Mexican–American families lack adequate access, health care providers remain an important and trusted source of information and guidance. The impact of health care in motivating positive nutrition and physical activity behaviors can be enhanced by the following actions:

- Develop guidelines outlining best practices for health care providers to assist in counseling Mexican–American youth and families regarding healthful dietary and physical activity habits. Anticipatory guidance by health care providers should begin early and include information on maternal nutrition, breastfeeding, infant nutrition, and healthful diet and physical activity for children, youth, and families.
- Provide health promotion materials and information that is adapted to Hispanic language and culture.
- Encourage the development and evaluation of training courses and materials for health care professionals in the assessment and behavioral management of child obesity, particularly when caring for Mexican–American children and adolescents.
- Encourage collaboration between medical, public health, and school services to provide consistent and thus reinforcing health promotion messages and support for populations of Mexican–American children who are at high risk for childhood obesity, independent of insurance status or ability to pay.

Research and Monitoring

Expanded research and evaluation efforts are needed to provide the scientific underpinnings for obesity prevention efforts. Priority areas for research and opportunities for Mexico–U.S. collaborations are outlined below.

- Establish policies to support behavioral research that can assess the impact of television, radio, Internet, and print media messages on eating habits and physical activity in Mexican–American children and youth.
- Conduct research on the use of the Internet by Hispanic families and children, especially when they are seeking health-related information. Segment by age, gender, income, education, and location.
- Conduct research on the effectiveness of Web-based health promotion directed at Mexican–American children and youth.
- Support research on the effectiveness of school-based interventions for obesity prevention, particularly relating to the impact on Mexican–American children and youth.
- Conduct research on the availability, use, and effectiveness of community-based health promotion activities for improving dietary choices and physical activity in Hispanic, especially Mexican–American, children and youth.
- Support research to better understand the attitudes and perceptions of Mexican Americans about the health consequences of obesity and the link between obesity and dietary and physical activity habits.
- Support continued monitoring of obesity prevalence and related risk factors at the national level, particularly in high-risk populations such as Mexican Americans.
- Support and expand state and local surveys that provide insight into obesity status, attitudes, and dietary and physical activity behaviors, especially in populations at increased risk.
- Facilitate interdisciplinary research between medicine, public health, architecture, planning, food production economics, and communication to explore the ecological model of childhood obesity, particularly relying on scholars from ethnic study centers.

Mexico–U.S. Collaboration

Achievement of goals for intervention, monitoring, and research of child and adolescent obesity will be assisted greatly by establishing a framework in which Mexican and United States' researchers, public health professionals, and policy makers can readily exchange ideas and information and can collaborate in future research and intervention efforts. Below are some specific steps that might be considered to foster such collaboration.

- Establish an ongoing mechanism for binational coordination to facilitate periodic meetings, e-mail newsletters, and other means of communication between Mexican and U.S. intervention program directors and researchers to exchange information on obesity prevention activities and research findings and to foster collaboration.

- Establish a Mexico–United States scientific exchange program that provides opportunities for researchers in obesity prevention to share ideas and undertake joint research.
- Identify specific intervention strategies that could be implemented and evaluated in both countries, such as
  - Use of a standardized health report card for tracking weight status and risk factors for obesity in children and youth,
  - Use of waist circumference as a screening tool to identify children and youth at risk,
  - Use of Internet-based resources (such as "todoenobesidad") to provide health information and guidance, and
  - Effectiveness of multicomponent school-based interventions to reduce behavioral and physiological risk factors, such as the Bienestar program.
- Develop a common framework for evaluating intervention effectiveness and provide opportunities, such as joint workshops, to review and learn from the experiences in each country.
- Provide awards that recognize significant research and programmatic accomplishments in obesity prevention relating to Mexican and Mexican–American children and youth.
- Provide training grants and fellowship support to encourage young researchers to enter the field of obesity prevention.
- Establish a Mexico–U.S. practice exchange that provides opportunities for public health, community organizations, advocates, policy makers, and others to share best practices, models, tools, and other information.
- Share and disseminate information on success stories in obesity prevention in both countries.

Advocacy

Learning from the experiences of other public health efforts, it is clear that success in obesity prevention will depend on the fostering of effective advocacy at many levels. As outlined in the *Accelerating Policy on Nutrition* report, the success of advocacy efforts will depend especially on accomplishing the following key objectives (Dorfman et al., 2005):

- Establish clear policy goals.
- Foster opportunities for dialog with a wide range of stakeholders to develop a common framework and terminology for describing the nature of the problem and the most effective means to achieve obesity prevention and to promote health.
- Seek political opportunities to advance the policy goals.

• Mobilize resources and invest in building infrastructure for advocacy, conducting research, and cultivating leadership.

REFERENCES

Action for Healthy Kids. 2005. *Events, Programs, and Reports.* [Online] Available: http://www.actionforhealthykids.org [accessed April 15, 2006].

Agredano Y, Schetzina K, Mendoza F. 2004. Are immigrant Mexican–American children at greater risk for asthma? *Pediatric Research* 1326.

Andersen R, Crespo C, Bartlett S, Cheskin L, Pratt M. 1998. Relationship of physical activity and television watching with body weight and level of fatness among children. *Journal of the American Medical Association* 279(12):938–942.

Babey S, Diamant A, Brown R, Hastert T. 2005. *California Adolescents Increasingly Inactive.* Los Angeles, CA: UCLA Center for Health Policy Research.

Bandura A. 1977. *Social Learning Theory.* Englewood Cliffs, NJ: Prentice Hall.

Bandura A. 1986. *Social Foundations of Thought and Action: A Social Cognitive Theory.* Englewood Cliffs, NJ: Prentice Hall.

Basiotis P, Carlson A, Gerrior S, Juan W, Lino M. 2004. The Healthy Eating Index, 1999–2000: Charting dietary patterns of Americans. *Family Economics and Nutrition Review* 16(1):39–48.

BLS (Bureau of Labor Statistics). 2004. *Comparison of Labor Force Participation Rates and the Age of Composition of Hispanic and White non-Hispanic Men. Employment Projections.* Washington, DC: U.S. Department of Labor.

Bowman SA, Gortmaker SL, Ebbeling CB, Pereira MA, Ludwig DS. 2004. Effect of fast-food consumption on energy intake and diet quality among children in a national household survey. *Pediatrics* 113(1):112–118.

Broadie M, Kjellson N, Hoff T, Parker M. 1999. Perception of Latinos, African Americans, and Whites on media as a health information source. *Howard Journal of Communication* 10(3):147–167.

Burgos A, Schetzina K, Dixon B, Mendoza F. 2005. Importance of generational status in examining access to and utilization of health care services by Mexican–American children. *Pediatrics* 115(3):e322–e330.

CDC (Centers for Disease Control and Prevention). 2003. Prevalence of diabetes and impaired fasting glucose in adults—United States 1999–2000. *Morbidity and Mortality Weekly Report* 52(35):833–837.

CDC. 2004. Trends in intake of energy and macronutrients—United States, 1971–2000. *Morbidity and Mortality Weekly Report* 53(4):80–82.

CDC. 2005a. *National Diabetes Fact Sheet.* [Online]. Available: http://www.diabetes.org/uedocuments/NationalDiabetes FactSheetRev.pdf [accessed November 10, 2006].

CDC. 2005b. *Prevalence of Overweight Among Children and Adolescents: United States 1999–2002.* [Online]. Available: http://www.cdc.gov/nchs/products/pubs/pubd/hestats/overwght99.htm. [accessed November 10, 2006].

CDC. 2005c. Public health strategies for preventing and controlling overweight and obesity in school and worksite settings: A report on recommendations of the Task Force on Community Preventive Services. *Morbidity and Mortality Weekly Report* 54(10):1–12. [Online]. Available: http://www.cdc.gov/MMWR/preview/mmwrhtml/rr5410a1.htm [accessed November 10, 2006].

CDC. 2006. *Physical and Mental Health Characteristics of U.S. and Foreign-Born Adults: United States, 1998–2003.* Advance Data from vital and health statistics No. 369. Hyattsville, MD: National Center for Health Statistics.

Chenoweth D. 2005. *The Economic Cost of Physical Inactivity, Obesity, and Overweight in California Adults: Health Care, Workers Compensation, and Loss Productivity.* New Bern, NC: Chenoweth and Associates, Inc.

Cole TJ, Bellizzi MC, Flegal KM, Dietz WH. 2000. Establishing a standard definition for child overweight and obesity worldwide: International Survey. *British Medical Journal* 320(7244):1240–1243.

Cruz ML, Weigensberg MJ, Huang TT, Ball G, Shaibi GQ, Goran MI. 2004. The metabolic syndrome in overweight Hispanic youth and the role of insulin sensitivity. *Journal of Clinical Endocrinology and Metabolism* 89(1):108–113.

Daniels SR, Khoury PR, Morrison JA. 1997. The utility of body mass index as a measure of body fatness in children and adolescents: Differences by race and gender. *Pediatrics* 99(6):804–807.

Datar A, Magnabosco JL. 2004. Childhood overweight and academic performance: National study of kindergartners and first-graders. *Obesity Research* 12(1):58–68.

Davidson KK, Birch LL. 2001. Weight status, parental reaction and self-concept in five-year-old girls. *Pediatrics* 107(1):46–53.

del Rio-Navarro BE, Velazquez-Monroy O, Sanchez-Castillo CP, Lara-Esqueda A, Berber A, Fanghanel G, Violante R, Tapia-Conyer R, James W. 2004. The high prevalence of overweight and obesity in Mexican children. *Obesity Research* 12(2):215–223.

DeNavas-Walt C, Proctor B, Lee C. 2005. *Income, Poverty, and Health Insurance Coverage in the United States: 2004.* U.S. Census Bureau. Washington, DC: U.S. Department of Commerce.

Dixon LB, Sundquist J, Winkleby M. 2000. Differences in energy, nutrient, and food intakes in a U.S. sample of Mexican American women and men: Findings from the third National Health and Nutrition Examination Survey, 1988–1994. *American Journal of Epidemiology* 152(6):548–557.

Dorfman L, Wilbur P, Lingas EO, Woodruff K, Wallack L. 2005 *Accelerating Policy on Nutrition: Lessons from Tobacco, Alcohol, Firearms, and Traffic Safety.* Final report from a series of meetings conducted by the Berkeley Media Studies Group. Oakland, CA: Public Health Institute.

Duke J, Huhman M, Heitzler C. 2003. Physical activity levels among children aged 9–13 years—United States 2002. *Morbidity and Mortality Weekly Report* 52(33):785–788.

Endicott RC, Brown K, MacDonald S, Schumann M, Ryan M, Sierra J, Wentz L. 2005. *Hispanic Pact Pack. Advertising Age* (Supplement). Pp. 1–51. [Online]. Available: http://www.adage.com/images/random/hispfactpack05.pdf.

Fernandez JR, Redden DT, Pietrobelli A, Allison DB. 2004. Waist circumference percentiles in nationally representative samples of African American, European American, and Mexican American children and adolescents. *Journal of Pediatrics* 145(4):439–444.

Finkelstein EA, Fiebelkorn IC, Wang G. 2004. State-level estimates of annual medical expenditures attributable to obesity. *Obesity Research* 12(1):18–24.

Flores G, Abreu M, Olivar MA, Kastner B. 1998. Access barriers to health care for Latino children. *Archives of Pediatrics and Adolescent Medicine* 152(11):1119–1125.

Food and Nutrition Service. 2005. *Making It Happen! School Nutrition Success Stories.* Alexandria, VA: U.S. Department of Health and Human Services, U.S. Department of Agriculture, and U.S. Department of Education.

Ford ES, Mokdad AH, Ajani UA. 2004. Trends in risk factors for cardiovascular disease among children and adolescents in the United States. *Pediatrics* 114(6):1534–1544.

Freedman DS, Dietz WH, Srinivasan SR, Berenson GS. 1999. The relation of overweight to cardiovascular risk factors among children and adolescents: The Bogalusa Heart Study. *Pediatrics* 103(6):1175–1182.

Freedman DS, Khan LK, Dietz WH, Srinivasan SR, Berenson GS. 2001. Relationship of childhood obesity to coronary heart disease risk factors in adulthood: The Bogalusa Heart Study. *Pediatrics* 108(3):712–718.

Freedman DS, Khan LK, Serdula MK, Galuska DA, Dietz WH. 2002. Trends and correlates of class 3 obesity in the United States from 1990 through 2000. *Journal of the American Medical Association* 288(14):1758–1761.

GAO (U.S. Government Accountability Office). 2005. *Childhood Obesity: Most Experts Identified Physical Activity and the Use of Best Practices as Key to Successful Programs.* GAO-06-127R. Washington, DC: GAO.

Gribble LS, Falciglia G, Davis AM, Couch SC. 2003. A curriculum based on social learning theory emphasizing fruit exposure and positive parent child-feeding strategies: A pilot study. *Journal of the American Dietetic Association* 103(1):100–103.

Hammer L. 2005. *Personal communication.* Stanford, CA: Medical Director, Center for Health Weight.

Hannon TS, Rao G, Arslanian SA. 2005. Childhood obesity and type 2 diabetes mellitus. *Pediatrics* 116(2):473–480.

Hayden-Wade HA, Stein RI, Ghaderi A, Saelens BE, Zabinski MF, Wilfley DE. 2005. Prevalence, characteristics, and correlates of teasing experiences among overweight children vs. non-overweight peers. *Obesity Research* 13(8):1381–1392.

Heath EM, Coleman KJ. 2002. Evaluation of the institutionalization of the Coordinated Approach to Child Health (CATCH) in a U.S./Mexico border community. *Health Education and Behavior* 29(4):444–460.

Hedley AA, Ogden CL, Johnson CL, Carroll MD, Flegal KM. 2004. Prevalence of overweight and obesity among U.S. children, adolescents, and adults. *Journal of the American Medical Association* 91(23):2847–2850.

Hernandez D. 2004. Children of immigrant families: Demographic changes and the life circumstances of immigrant families. *The Future of Children* 14(2):17–47.

Huhman M, Potter LD, Wong FL, Banspach SW, Duke JC, Heitzler CD. 2005. Effects of a mass media campaign to increase physical activity among children: Year-1 results of the VERB campaign. *Pediatrics* 116(2):e277–e284.

International Life Sciences Institute. 2005. ILSI CHP *Nutrition and Physical Activity Program List.* [Online]. Available: http://chp.ilsi.org/Publications/CHPPhysicalActivityProgram List.htm [accessed April 15, 2006].

IOM (Institute of Medicine). 2005. *Preventing Childhood Obesity: Health in the Balance.* Washington, DC: The National Academies Press.

IOM. 2006. *Food Marketing to Children and Youth: Threat or Opportunity?* Washington, DC: The National Academies Press.

Kahn HS, Imperatore G, Cheng YJ. 2005. A population-based comparison of BMI percentiles and waist-to-height ratio for identifying cardiovascular risk in youth. *Journal of Pediatrics* 146(4):482–488.

Kaplan MS, Huguet N, Newsom JT, McFarland BH. 2004. The association between length of residence and obesity among Hispanic immigrants. *American Journal of Preventive Medicine* 27(4):323–326.

Kaplowitz H, Martorell R, Mendoza F. 1989. Fatness and fat distribution in Mexican American children and youth from the Hispanic Health and Nutrition Examination Survey. *American Journal of Human Biology* 1:631–648.

Katzmarzyk PT, Srinivasan SR, Chen W, Malina RM, Bouchard C, Berenson GS. 2004. Body mass index, waist circumference, and clustering of cardiovascular disease risk factors in a biracial sample of children and adolescents. *Pediatrics* 114:e198–e205.

Kissam E, Intili J, Garcia A. 2003. Spanish-Language community radio as a resource for health promotion campaigns targeted to farmworkers and recent immigrants. *Californian Journal of Health Promotion* 1(2):183–197.

Klaudt M, Schetzina K, Mendoza F, Robinson T. 2002. *Racial/Ethnic Differences in Maternal Perception of Children's Weight.* Ambulatory Pediatric Association, Region IX and X, February 2002 Annual Meeting. Carmel, CA.

Kovacs P, Ma L, Hanson RL, Franks P, Stumvoll M, Bogardus C, Baier LJ. 2005. Genetic variation in UCP 2 (uncoupling protein 2) is associated with energy metabolism in Pima Indians. *Diabetologia* 48(11):2292–2295.

Kuczmarski RJ, Ogden CL, Guo SS. 2002. 2000 CDC growth charts for the United States: Methods and development. National Center for Health Statistics. *Vital Health Statistics* 11:246.

Li X, Li S, Ulusoy E, Chen W, Srinivasan SR, Berenson GS. 2004. Childhood adiposity as a predictor of cardiac mass in adulthood: The Bogalusa Heart Study. *Circulation* 110(22):3488–3492.

López R, Barquera S, Hernandez Prado B, Rivera JR. 2006. *Preventing Obesity in Mexican Children and Adolescents.* U.S.–Mexico Workshop on Prevention of Childhood Obesity. Washington, DC: Institute of Medicine.

Malina R, Martorell R, Mendoza F. 1986. Growth status of Mexican American children and youth: Historical trends and contemporary issues. *American Journal of Physical Anthropology* 29(S7):45–79.

Martorell R, Mendoza FS, Castillo RO, Pawson IG, Budge CC. 1987. Short and plump physique of Mexican American children. *American Journal of Physical Anthropology* 73:475–478.

Martorell R, Malina RM, Castillo RO, Mendoza FS, Pawson IG. 1988a. Body proportions in three ethnic groups: Children and youths 2–17 years in NHANES II and HHANES. *Human Biology* 60(2):205–222.

Martorell R, Mendoza F, Castillo R. 1988b. Poverty and stature in children. In: *Linear Growth Retardation in Less Developed Countries.* Waterlow JC. Ed. New York: Raven Press 14:57–73.

Martorell R, Mendoza F, Castillo R. 1989. Genetic and environmental determinants of growth in Mexican Americans. *Pediatrics* 84(5):864–871.

Maynard MG, Blanck H, Serdula M. 2003. Maternal perception of weight status of children. *Pediatrics* 111:1226–1231.

Mazur RE, Marquis GS, Jensen HH. 2003. Diet and food insufficiency among Hispanic youth: Acculturation and socioeconomic factors in the third National Health and Nutrition Examination Survey. *American Journal of Clinical Nutrition* 78:1120–1127.

Mendoza F, Castillo R. 1986. Growth abnormalities in Mexican–American children in the United States: The NHANES I Study. *Nutrition Research* 6:1247–1257.

Morrison JA, Friedman LA, Harlan WR, Harlan LC, Barton BA, Schreiber GB, Klein DJ. 2005. Development of the metabolic syndrome in black and white adolescent girls: A longitudinal assessment. *Pediatrics* 116(5):1178–1182.

Murphy S, Castillo R, Martorell R, Mendoza F. 1990. An evaluaiton of the food group intakes by Mexican American children. *Journal of the American Dietetic Association* 90(3): 388–393.

Nader MD, Stone EJ, Lytle LA, Perry CL, Osganian SK, Kelder S, Webber LS, Elder JP, Montgomery D, Feldman HA, Wu M, Johnson C, Parcel GS, Luepker RV. 1999. Three-year maintenance of improved diet and physical activity. *Archives of Pediatrics and Adolescent Medicine* 153(7):695–704.

Narayan KM, Boyle JP, Thompson TJ, Sorensen SW, Williamson DF. 2003. Lifetime risk for diabetes mellitus in the United States. *Journal of the American Medical Association* 290(14):1884–1890.

NCHS (National Center for Health Statistics). 2004. *Health, United States, 2004, with Chartbook on Trends in the Health of Americans.* Hyattsville, MD: NCHS.

Neufeld ND, Raffel LJ, Landon C, Chen YD, Vadheim C. 1998. Early presentation of type 2 diabetes in Mexican American youth. *Diabetes Care* 21(1):80–86.

Neuhouser ML, Thompson B, Coronado GD, Solomon CC. 2004. Higher fat intake and lower fruit and vegetables intakes are associated with greater acculturation among Mexicans living in Washington State. *Journal of the American Dietetic Association* 104(1):51–57.

NRC/IOM (National Research Council/Institute of Medicine). 1998. *From Generation to Generation: The Health and Well-Being of Children in Immigrant Families.* Washington, DC: National Academy Press.

NRC/IOM. 1999. *Children of Immigrants: Health, Adjustment, and Public Assistance.* Washington, DC: National Academy Press. Pp. 187–243.

Ogden CL, Flegal KM, Carroll MD, Johnson CL. 2002. Prevalence and trends in overweight among United States children and adolescents, 1999–2000. *Journal of the American Medical Association* 288(14):1728–1732.

Ogden CL, Carroll MD, Curtin LR, McDowell MA, Tabak CJ, Flegal KM. 2006. Prevalence of overweight and obesity in the United States, 1999–2004. *Journal of the American Medical Association* 288295(13):1549–1555.

Olaiz G, Rojas R, Barquera S, Shamah T, Aguilar C, Cravioto P, López P, Hernández M, Tapia R, Sepúlveda J. 2003. *Encuesta Nacional de Salud 2000.* Tomo 2. La salud de los adultos. Cuernavaca, Morelos, México: Instituto Nacional de Salud Pública.

Pelayo R. 2005. Personal communication. Palo Alto, CA: Stanford Sleep Center.

Pietrobelli A, Faith MS, Allison DB, Gallagher D, Chiumello G, Heymsfield SB. 1998. Body mass index as a measure of adiposity among children and adolescents: A validation study. *Journal of Pediatrics* 132(2):204–210.

Pinhas-Hamiel O, Dolan LM, Daniels SR, Standiford D, Khoury PR, Zeitler P. 1996. Increased incidence of non-insulin dependent diabetes mellitus among adolescents. *Journal of Pediatrics* 128:608–615.

Popkin B, Udry JR. 1998. Adolescent obesity increases significantly in second and third generation U.S. immigrants: The national longitudinal study of adolescent health. *Journal of Nutrition* 128:701–706.

Reaven P, Nader PR, Berry C, Hoy T. 1998. Cardiovascular disease insulin risk in Mexican–American and Anglo-American children and mothers. *Pediatrics* 101(4):1–7.

Rivera J, Shamah Levy T, Villalpando Hernández S, González de Cossío T, Hernández Prado B, Sepúlveda J. 2001. *Encuesta Nacional de Nutrición 1999.* Estado nutricio de niños y mujeres en México. Cuernavaca, Morelos, México: Instituto Nacional de Salud Pública.

Rivera JA, Barquera S, Campirano F, Campos I, Safdie M, Tovar V. 2002. Epidemiological and nutritional transition in Mexico: Rapid increase of non-communicable chronic diseases and obesity. *Public Health Nutrition* 5(1A):113–122.

Roberts DF, Foehr UG, Rideout V. 2005. *Generation M: Media in the Lives of 8–18 Year Olds.* KFF. [Online]. Available: http://www.kff.org/entmedia/upload/Generation-M-Media-in-the-Lives-of-8-18-Year-olds-Report.pdf [accessed April 15, 2006].

Romero A, Robinson T, Haydel K, Mendoza F, Killen J. 2004. Association among familism, language preference, and education in Mexican American mothers and their children. *Journal of Developmental and Behavioral Pediatrics* 25(1):34–40.

Ryan AS, Roche AF, Kuczmarski RJ. 1999. Weight, stature, and body mass index data for Mexican Americans from the third national health and nutrition examination survey. *American Journal of Human Biology* 11:673–686.

Salsberry PJ, Reagan PB. 2005. Dynamics of early childhood overweight. *Pediatrics* 116(6):1329.

Sanchez-Castillo CP, Lara JJ, Villa AR, Aguirre J, Escobar M, Gutierrez H, Chavez A, James WP. 2005. Unusually high prevalence rates of obesity in four Mexican rural communities. *Public Health Nutrition* 8(1):53–60.

Schwimmer JB, Burwinkle TM, Varni J. 2003. Health-related quality of life of severely obese children and adolescents. *Journal of the American Medical Association* 289(14):1813–1819.

Shaping America's Youth. 2004. *Shaping America's Youth.* [Online]. Available: http://www.shapingamericasyouth.org/Programs.aspx?page=search [accessed April 15, 2006].

Siegel JM, Yancey AK, Aneshensel CS, Schuler R. 1999. Body image, perceived pubertal timing and adolescent mental health. *Journal of Adolescent Health* 25(2):155–165.

Spooner T, Rainie L. 2001. *Hispanics and the Internet. Pew Internet and American Life Project.* [Online]. Available: http://www.pewinternet.org/PPF/r/38/report_display.asp [accessed April 15, 2006].

Srinivasan SR, Myers L, Berenson GS. 2002. Predictability of childhood adiposity and insulin for developing Insulin Resistance Syndrome (Syndrome X) in young adulthood: The Bogalusa Heart Study. *Diabetes* 51:204–209.

Strauss RS, Pollack HA. 2001. Epidemic increase in childhood overweight, 1986–1998. *Journal of the American Medical Association* 286(22):2845.

Strohl KP, Redline S. 1996. Recongition of obstructive sleep apnea. *American Journal of Respiratory and Critical Care Medicine* 154:279–289.

Thorpe KE, Florence CS, Howard DH, Joski P. 2004. The impact of obesity on rising medical spending. *Health Affairs*. Web Exclusive. October 20:W4-480 to W4-486.

Trevino RP, Hernandez A, Hale DE, Garcia OA, Mobley C. 2005. Impact of the Bienestar school-based diabetes mellitus prevention program on fasting capillary glucose levels: A randomized controlled trial. *Archives of Pediatrics and Adolescent Medicine* 158(9):911–917.

Trevino RP, Pugh JA, Hernandez AE, Menchaca VD, Ramirez RR, Mendoza M. 1998. Bienestar: A diabetes risk-factor prevention program. *Journal of School Health* 68(2):62–67.

USPSTF (U.S. Preventive Service Task Force). 2002. *Physical Activity Counseling.* [Online]. Available: http://www.ahrq.gov/clinic/uspstf/uspsphys.htm [accessed April 15, 2006].

USPSTF. 2003. *Healthy Diet Counseling.* [Online]. Available: http://www.ahrq.gov/clinic/uspstf/uspsdiet.htm [accessed April 15, 2006].

Velez-Subervi F. 1999. Spanish-language television coverage of health news. *Howard Journal of Communications* 10(3):207–228.

Wang G, Dietz WH. 2002. Economic burden of obesity in youths aged 6–17 years. *Pediatrics* 109(5):e81–e87.

Whitaker RC. 2004. Predicting preschooler obesity at birth: The role of maternal obesity in early pregnancy. *Pediatrics* 114(1):e29.

Whitlock EP, Williams SB, Gold R, Smith PR, Shipman SA. 2005. Screening and interventions for childhood overweight: A summary of evidence for the U.S. Preventive Services Task Force. *Pediatrics* 116(1):e125–e144.

Williams DE, Cadwell BL, Cheng YJ, Cowie CC, Gregg EW, Geiss LS, Engelgau MM, Narayan KM, Imperatore G. 2005. Prevalence of impaired fasting glucose and its relationship with cardiovascular disease risk factors in U.S. adolescents, 1999–2000. *Pediatrics* 116(5):1122–1126.

Yusuf S, Hawken S, Ounpuu S, Bautista L, Franzosi MG, Commerford P, Lang CC, Rumboldt Z, Onen CL, Lisheng L, Tanomsup S, Wangai P Jr, Razak F, Sharma AM, Anand SS, INTERHEART Study Investigators. 2005. Obesity and the risk of myocardial infarction in 27,000 participants from 52 countries: A case-control study. *Lancet* 366(9497):1640–1649.

D

Workshop Participants

Dr. Reynaldo Martorell *(Chair)*
Robert W. Woodruff Professor of Public Health, and Chair, Department of Global Health
Rollins School of Public Health
Emory University
Atlanta, GA

Dr. Jeffrey Koplan
Vice President for Academic Health Affairs
Woodruff Health Sciences Center
Emory University
Atlanta, GA

Dr. Juan Rivera Dommarco
Director, Nutrition and Health Research Center
National Institute of Public Health
Col. Santa María Ahuacatitlán
Morelos, México

Lic. Guillermo Ayala Alvarez
Director de Salud y seguridad en las Escuelas
Dirección General de Innovación y Fortalecimiento Académico SEP
México, D.F.

Dr. Eduardo García Anaya
Coordinador del Departamento de la Clínica y Obesidad y Trastornos Alimenticios
Instituto Nacional de Ciencias Médicas y Nutrición "Dr. Salvador Zubirán"
Vasco de Quiroga
México

Dr. Mauricio Hernández Ávila
Director General
Instituto Nacional de Salud Pública
Santa Maria Ahuacatitlán
Cuernavaca, Morelos
México

Dr. Simón Barquera
Jefe de departamento de Nutrición y Enfermedades Crónicas
Cuernavaca, Morelos
México

Ing. José Luis Prado Becerra
Presidente de Grupo Gamesa
Agustín, Garza García Nuevo León
México

Dr. Diana M. Bonta
Vice President, Public Affairs
Kaiser Permanente
Southern California Region
Pasadena, CA

Dr. Xochitl Casteneda
Director
California-Mexico Health Initiative
University of California, Berkeley
Berkeley, CA

Lic. Rolando Arreola Castillo
Director
General de Educación Física, SEP
México

Lic. Enrique de la Madrid Cordero
Presidente
CONMEXICO y Diputado Federal
Consejo Mexicano de la Industria de Productos de Consumo, A.C.
México, D.F.

Ms. Camila Corvalan
Ph.D. student
Nutrition and Health Sciences Program
Emory University
Atlanta, GA

Dr. Arturo Jiménez Cruz
Profesor de la Facultad de Medicina
Universidad Autónoma de Baja California
Tijuana Baja California
México

Dr. Esteban Cruz
Kaiser Permanente
110 North La Brea Ave.
Inglewood, CA 90301

Dra. Teresa Gonzalez de Cossio
Investigador del CINYS
Cuernavaca Morelos
México

Dr. Agustín Lara Esqueda
Director del Programa de Salud del Adulto y el Anciano.
Centro Nacioanal de Vigilancia
Epidemiológica y Control de Enfermedades
México

Dr. Lance Friedmann
Senior Vice President, Global Health and Wellness and New Category Development
Kraft Foods, Inc.
Northfield State, IL

Lic. Luis Alfonso Caso González
Comisionado de Fomento Sanitario
Comisión Federal para la Protección contra Riesgos Sanitarios
México

Dr. Juan Manuel Hernández
Director del Programa de Atención de la Salud de la Infancia y la Adolescencia
Centro Nacional para la Salud de la Infancia y la Adolescencia SSA
México

Dr. Eileen Kennedy
Dean
Friedman School of Nutrition Science and Policy
Tufts University
Boston, MA 02111

Dr. Laura Kettel Khan
Deputy Chief
Chronic Disease Nutrition Division of Nutrition and Physical Activity
National Center for Chronic Disease Prevention and Health Promotion
Atlanta, GA

Ms. Vivica Kraak
Senior Program Officer
Food and Nutrition Board
Institute of Medicine
The National Academies
Washington, DC

Dr. Marinela Servitje de Lerdo de Tejada
Directora
Papalote Museo del Niño
Col. Daniel Garza
México, D.F.

Dr. Amy Luke
Associate Professor
Department of Preventive Medicine and Epidemiology/Family Medicine
Loyola University School of Medicine
Maywood, IL

Dr. Marcella Martinez
Deputy Director of Constituency Services
National Association of Latino Elected and Appointed Officials (NALEO) Educational Fund
Los Angeles, CA 90015

Dr. J. Armando Barriguette Meléndez
Presidente de la Fundación Franco-Mexicana para la Medicina IAP
Col. Guadalupe Inn
México, D.F.

Dr. Fernando Mendoza
Professor of Pediatrics
Department of Pediatrics
Stanford University School of Medicine
Palo Alto, CA

Dr. Jorge A. Meyer
Vice President
Corporate Affairs and International Trade
Department of Corporate Affairs
Institutional Communications, Public Relations, and Government and Regulatory Affairs
Sabritas Region of PepsiCo International
Mexico, D.F.

Dr. Linda D. Meyers
Director
Food and Nutrition Board
Institute of Medicine
The National Academies
Washington, DC

Dr. Julio Frenk Mora
Secretario de Salud
Lieja No. 7 1er Piso
Col Juárez
México, D.F.

Dr. Carmen Rita Nevarez
Medical Director and VP of External Relations
Public Health Institute
Oakland, CA

Dr. Nancy Nieves-Cruz
Doctor of Internal Medicine
Childhood Obesity Team
The Robert Wood Johnson Foundation
Princeton, NJ

Arq. Fernando Padres Oelrich
Presidente
Asociación Mexicana de Urbanismo
Col. Cuajimalpa, Deleg. Cuajimalpa
México

Dr. Maria Oria
Senior Program Officer
Food and Nutrition Board
Institute of Medicine
The National Academies
Washington, DC

Dr. Russell Pate
Professor
Department of Exercise Science
Arnold School of Public Health
University of South Carolina
Columbia, SC

Dr. Bernardo Hernández Prado
Director del Área de Salud Reproductiva
Cuernavaca, Morelos
México

Dr. Patrick Racsa
Data Analyst
Friedman School of Nutrition Science and Policy
Tufts University
Boston, MA

Dr. Ruy López Ridaura
Director del área de Enfermedades Crónicas.
Cuernavaca Morelos
México

Lic. Carmela Rivero
Presidente de Investigación y Desarrollo
de Sabritas
Centro de Tecnolgia
Sabritas
México, D.F.

Dr. Thomas N. Robinson
Associate Professor of Pediatrics and Medicine
Stanford Prevention Research Center
Stanford University School of Medicine
Hoover Pavilion
Stanford, CA

Dr. Martín Nacif Rojas
Secretario Técnico
Comisión de Salud de la Cámara de Diputados
México

Dr. Jaime Sepúlveda
Coordinador General de los Institutos Nacionales de Salud SSA
Del. Alvaro Obregón
México, D.F.

Dr. Rafael Camacho Solís
Encargado de la División de Bienestar Social IMSS
Col. Cuauhtémoc
México, D.F.

Dr. Frederick Trowbridge
President
Trowbridge & Associates, Inc.
Decatur, GA

Dr. Robert Otto Valdez
Chief Health Advisor
Univision's "Salud es Vida: Enterate!"
President, Valdez & Associates
Senior Health Scientist, RAND

Dr. Heladio Gerardo Verver y Vargas
Director General de Servicios de Salud de Zacatecas
Av. Gónzalez Ortega Esq. Dr. Castro
Zacatecas
México

Sen. Marco Antonio Xicotencatl
Grupo Parlamanetario del PAN
Del. Cuauhtemoc C.P 06600
México, D.F.

E

Speakers' Biographies

Bernardo Hernández, Ph.D., is a National Researcher Level I of the National System of Researchers-Mexico. He is also a Senior Researcher "E" at the Research Center in Populational Health, National Institute of Public Health (INSP). His areas or interest are reproductive health (especially maternal mortality), evaluation of social and health programs, physical activity, and obesity. Dr. Hernández received his B.Sc. degree in Social Psychology at the Metropolitan Autonomous University-Mexico City, his Masters in Social Psychology at the London School of Economics (LSE), and his Doctorate in Sciences in Health and Social Behavior (Harvard School Public Health, HSPH).

Mauricio Hernández-Ávila, M.D., earned his MD degree from the National Autonomous University of Mexico (UNAM) in 1980. He has a master's degree in statistics from UNAM Applied Mathematics and Systems Research Institute (1984). He also holds a Master of Public Health degree (1984) and a Ph.D. in Epidemiology (1988), both from the Harvard School of Public Health. Dr. Hernández has participated in several international health committees, including "Lead in the Americas: Strategies for Disease Prevention" and "Physicians for Social Responsibility U.S.-Mexico Border Environmental Health Task Force". In 1996, he received the Miguel Aleman Award in the area of health. Dr. Hernández is the author of 199 published scientific articles and 7 articles for diffusion, and has written 6 books and 45 chapters of books. He has mentored and trained six doctoral students in the area of epidemiology and has been invited to more than 178 scientific events, both national and international. He built an inter-institutional team called the Environmental Health Unit dedicated to environmental health research, and as the leader of this group he has produced a large number of scientific articles in the area of lead poison. Dr. Hernández is a researcher of national and international prestige. He has been a member of the National Academy of Medicine since 1993 and of the National System of Researchers (Level III National Investigator) since 1990. He also sits on the Committee of Biomedical Sciences of CONACyT.

Jeffrey P. Koplan, M.D., M.P.H., is Vice President for Academic Health Affairs of Emory University's Woodruff Health Sciences Center. In this position, he is responsible for coordination and oversight of academic matters including research and education in Emory's schools of medicine, nursing, and public health and the Yerkes National Primate Research Center. From 1998 to 2002, Dr. Koplan served as the Director of the Centers for Disease Control and Prevention (CDC). Dr. Koplan began his public health career in the early 1970s as one of the CDC's celebrated "disease detectives," more formally known as Epidemic Intelligence Service (EIS) Officers. Since then, he has worked on virtually every major public health issue, including infectious diseases such as smallpox and HIV/AIDS, environmental issues such as the Bhopal chemical disaster, and the health toll of tobacco and chronic diseases, both in the United States and around the globe. He recently chaired the Institute of Medicine committee on preventing childhood obesity and is internationally active in promoting healthy nutrition and physical activity. From 1994 to 1998, he pursued his interest in enhancing the interactions between clinical medicine and public health by leading the Prudential Center for Health Care Research, a nationally recognized health services research organization. Dr. Koplan is a graduate of Yale College, the Mt. Sinai School of Medicine, and the Harvard School of Public Health. He is a Master of the American College of Physicians and was elected to membership in the Institute of Medicine, where he was elected to the Governing Council. He has served on many advisory groups and consultancies in the U.S. and overseas, and has written more than 190 scientific papers. He is a trustee of Yale University, The Marcus Family Foundation, HealthMPowers, and Kaiser Foundation Health Plan of Georgia, Inc.

Ruy López is Chief of the Chronic Disease Division of the Population and Health Research Center at the National Institute of Public Health, Mexico. He has an M.D., Residency in Internal Medicine, and M.Sc. from the National University of Mexico and an Sc.D. candidate in Nutritional Epidemiology from Harvard University. His research and publications have focused on the genetic and dietary determinants of diabetes mellitus and related conditions such as metabolic syndrome and cardiovascular disease. Since his incorporation at the National Institute of Public Health in Mexico, he is coordinating several projects related to the diabetes and obesity epidemics in Mexico, focusing on individual and collective determinants, specifically dietary and lifestyle factors related to the transition occurring in Mexico.

Reynaldo Martorell, Ph.D., is the Robert W. Woodruff Professor of Public Health and Chair of the Hubert Department of Global Health, Rollins School of Public Health, Emory University. Previously, he was Leading Professor, Division of Nutritional Sciences, Cornell University and Professor of Nutrition, Food Research Institute, Stanford University. He began his career at the Division of Human Development, Institute of Nutrition of Central America and Panama (INCAP) in Guatemala. Dr. Martorell's research interests include maternal and child nutrition (particularly in developing countries), child growth and development, the significance of early childhood malnutrition for short- and long-term human function, micronutrient malnutrition, and the emergence of obesity and chronic diseases in developing countries. Dr. Martorell's policy interests include global health concerns, particularly programs and policies in food and nutrition, issues dealing with hunger and malnutrition, and the health implications of changes in diet and lifestyles in developing countries (including the emergence of obesity and related chronic diseases of dietary origin in developing countries). He has been a member of several IOM committees and currently serves on the Food and Nutrition Board. Dr. Martorell is a consultant to the World Bank, UNICEF, and WHO and a board member of the International Nutrition Foundation for Developing Countries and the Pan American Health and Education Foundation. Dr. Martorell received a Bachelor degree in Anthropology from St. Louis University and a Ph.D. in Biological Anthropology from the University of Washington. He was elected to the Institute of Medicine in 2002.

Fernando Sanchez Mendoza, M.D., M.P.H., is Professor and Chief of the Division of General Pediatrics at the Lucile Packard Children's Hospital at Stanford and Associate Dean for Minority Advising and Programs at Stanford University School of Medicine. Dr. Mendoza received his undergraduate degree from San Jose State College, his medical degree from Stanford University, and did his pediatric residency at Stanford University Hospital. After residency, he obtained a Master of Public Health degree from Harvard University, and then returned to Stanford as a Robert Wood Johnson Academic General Pediatric Fellow. Dr. Mendoza's research interests have focused on Hispanic children's health. He has published numerous articles and chapters on the growth and health status of Mexican–

American children and is a national expert in the field. He is a reviewer for a number of scientific journals and served on the National Institutes of Health, Human Development and Aging Study Section. He was a member of the Institute of Medicine's Committee on the Health and Adjustment of Immigrant Children and Families, and authored a report on the health and nutrition of immigrant Hispanic children. His current work focuses on childhood obesity in Hispanic children. As Associate Dean for Minority Advising and Programs, Dr. Mendoza has been involved in the career development of minority medical students and faculty both at Stanford Medical School and at the national level as past President of the Hispanic Serving Health Professions School Inc. He is a fellow of the Academy of Pediatrics, a member of the Ambulatory Pediatric Association, and the American Pediatric Society, and is listed in the "Best Doctors in America." Dr. Mendoza has received a number of awards for his service to the Hispanic community, and *Hispanic Business Magazine* has named him as among the 100 most influential Hispanics in the United States.

Juan A. Rivera, Ph.D., is the founding Director of the Center for Research in Nutrition and Health at the National Institute of Public Health and is a Professor of Nutrition in the School of Public Health in Mexico. He is also an adjunct professor at Cornell University and the Rollins School of Public Health at Emory University. Dr. Rivera earned both his master's and doctorate degrees from Cornell University in International Nutrition with minors in Epidemiology and Statistics. Dr. Rivera is a former director of Nutrition and Health at the Nutrition Institute of Central America and Panama (INCAP). He is the co-chair of the International Zinc Nutrition Consultative Group (IZiNCG). Since 2000, he's been a member of the panel of experts of the World Cancer Research Fund (WCRF) and has been appointed to the National Academy of Medicine and to the Mexican Academy of Sciences in Mexico. He was a member of the board of the International Union of Nutritional Scientists (IUNS) from 2001 to 2005 and of the Global Alliance for Improved Nutrition (GAIN) Board until 2005. He is the Chair of the International Nutrition Council of the American Society for Nutrition. Dr. Rivera has published more than 130 scientific articles, book chapters, and books, and is currently a member of the Latin American Nutrition Society, the American Society for Nutritional Sciences, and the Society for International Nutrition Research. His research interests include the epidemiology of stunting, the short- and long-term effects of undernutrition during early childhood, the effects of zinc and other micronutrient deficiencies on growth and health, the study of malnutrition in Mexico, and the design and evaluation of programs to improve nutritional status of children.

Jaime Sepúlveda, M.D., Dr.Sc., is Director General of the National Institutes of Health (NIH) of Mexico. He was appointed by President Fox in November 2003. As Director, he is responsible for setting policy; planning and coordinating the programs and activities of 12 NIH institutes; and overseeing an intra-mural operational budget of almost US $1 billion. Prior to this appointment, Dr. Sepúlveda was elected Director General of the National Institute of Public Health (INSP)—1 of the 12 NIH institutes in 1995, and reelected to a second term in 2000. During this time, he also served as the Dean of the National School of Public Health (NSPH), the first and most prestigious school in Latin America founded in 1922. As Director General of Epidemiology (1985–1991) and Vice-Minister of Health (1991–1994), he strengthened the country's Epidemiologic Surveillance System and founded a Universal Vaccination Program, which increased coverage for preschool vaccination from 45 to 94 percent in two years, and successfully eliminated poliomyelitis and diphtheria from Mexico. He was elected and currently serves on the Harvard Board of Overseers (2002–2008), which is one of the two governing boards of the university. He was also elected to the Institute of Medicine in 2004 and currently serves as chair to the IOM Committee responsible for evaluating the implementation of the U.S. President's Emergency Plan for AIDS Relief (PEPFAR). Dr. Sepúlveda earned his Medical Degree at the National Autonomous University of Mexico (UNAM) in 1978, followed by a Masters in Public Health in 1980, a Masters of Science in Tropical Medicine in 1981, and a Doctorate in Population Science in 1985, all from the Harvard School of Public Health.

Frederick Trowbridge, M.D., is President of Trowbridge & Associates, Inc. and has an extensive background in public health and nutrition issues, both in the United States and internationally. After completing clinical training and Board Certification in Pediatrics and a Master of Science degree in Human Nutrition, Dr. Trowbridge served for 25 years as a medical epidemiologist at the Centers for Disease Control and Prevention (CDC), assigned to the CDC Tropical Disease Research Station in El Salvador, the Johns Hopkins School of Hygiene and Public Health, and the Division of Nutrition and Physical Activity in Atlanta, where he served as Director for more than a decade. After retiring from CDC in 1996, Dr. Trowbridge served as Executive Director of the Nutrition and Health Promotion Program of the International Life Sciences Institute in Atlanta before founding Trowbridge & Associates, Inc. in 1998. Dr. Trowbridge is actively involved in research and in a wide range of consulting activities, particularly on topics relating to child and adolescent obesity, assessment of body weight status, and promotion of healthful dietary and physical activity behaviors in children and families. Recognizing the growing need for tools to assist healthcare professionals in the assessment and management of child obesity, Dr. Trowbridge recently developed the BMI Wheel, a CD-sized circular calculator that quickly computes body mass index in children, adolescents, or adults. Fluent in Spanish, Dr. Trowbridge has been particularly involved with health promotion efforts directed towards Hispanic populations.